FOOD
STANDARDS
AGENCY

Manual of Nutrition

Eleventh Edition

London: TSO

Published by TSO (The Stationery Office) and available from:

Online
www.tsoshop.co.uk

Mail, Telephone, Fax & E-mail
TSO
PO Box 29, Norwich, NR3 1GN
Telephone orders/General enquiries: 0870 600 5522
Fax orders: 0870 600 5533
E-mail: customer.services@tso.co.uk
Textphone 0870 240 3701

TSO Shops
16 Arthur Street, Belfast BT1 4GD
028 9023 8451 Fax 028 9023 5401
71 Lothian Road, Edinburgh EH3 9AZ
0870 606 5566 Fax 0870 606 5588

TSO@Blackwell and other Accredited Agents

Published with the permission of the Food Standards Agency on
behalf of the Controller of Her Majesty's Stationery Office.

Eleventh Edition 2008

ISBN 978 0 11 243116 9
Printed in the United Kingdom by the Stationery Office
N5734771 C50 05/08

Contents

PART 2: NUTRITIONAL VALUE OF FOOD AND DIETS

10   Introduction, and general effects of preparation and processing

11   Foods

List of Tables

Foreword

The eleventh edition of the *Manual of Nutrition* is published at a time when there has never been a greater public interest in the relationship between food and health. It is also a period of unprecedented efforts to tackle food-related public health problems such as cardiovascular disease, and the ever-increasing incidence of over weight and obesity in all age groups of the population. There is particular concern about saturated fat, salt and sugar intakes, but the science of nutrition is much broader than that. This manual therefore describes the major nutrients, their roles in the body, the foods that provide them, and the way in which these foods are digested so that the nutrients can be utilised by the body.

This edition covers similar ground to the previous edition, but contains the available values for the typical nutrient content of commonly eaten foods[1] as well as the nutrient intake of the population as estimated from Government surveys. A new feature is coverage of the safety aspects of vitamin and mineral intakes from dietary supplements, which were not available when the previous edition was published.

Reflecting current emphasis in dietary advice, new values for children's target salt intakes are included as are practical aids to achieving a healthy diet such as portion sizes for fruit and vegetables.

The Manual continues to be a valuable source of reference to a wide range of students, teachers and health professionals as well as interested members of the public as it was when the very first edition was produced sixty years ago.
This edition was prepared by Jennifer Woolfe who is grateful to all those who contributed in its preparation - Gillian Swan, Melanie Farron-Wilson, Louis Levy, Samantha Montel, Orla Hugueniot, Rufina Acheampong, Henry Odeje and Jamie Blackshaw.

Food Standards Agency

---

[1] Data available at the time of writing

PART 1

Nutrients and their utilization

1 Introduction to nutrition, and some definitions

Most people grow well and stay healthy provided that they get enough of a variety of foods to eat, wherever they live in the world. The reasons for this, and the ways in which the adequacy of any diet can be assessed, form part of the science of nutrition with which this manual is concerned. A knowledge of nutrition principles is therefore important to all of us, whether we plan and provide meals for ourselves and our families, cater for large numbers of customers or for vulnerable groups like older people, children or the sick, provide advice about healthier eating or teach nutrition to children at school.

Before proceeding further, it is necessary to define some terms:

The science of *nutrition* is the study of all processes of growth, maintenance and repair of the living body which depend upon the digestion of food, and the study of that food.

Food is any solid or liquid which when swallowed can supply any of the following:

(a) material from which the body can produce movement, heat or other forms of energy
(b) material for growth, repair or reproduction
(c) substances necessary to regulate the production of energy or the processes of growth and repair.

Foods are considered in more detail in Part 2.

The components of foods which have these functions are called *nutrients*. They are introduced below, and considered in more detail in Chapters 2, 3, 4, 7 and 8. The *diet* consists of those foods or mixtures of foods in the amounts which are actually eaten over the course of a week or so. A good diet provides adequate amounts of all the nutrients, without harmful excesses, from a wide range of foods.

The nutrients in food

The following types of nutrients may be present in foods:

Carbohydrates, which provide the body with energy; excess may also be converted into body fat.

Fats, which provide energy in a more concentrated form than carbohydrates, and may also be converted into body fat.

Proteins, which provide materials (amino acids) for growth and repair. They can also be converted into carbohydrate and used to provide energy.

As they are needed in relatively large quantities, carbohydrates, fats and proteins are sometimes referred to as macronutrients.

1

Minerals, which are used in growth and repair, and help to regulate body processes. *Vitamins*, which help to regulate body processes.[1]

Minerals and vitamins are needed in only small quantities and are sometimes referred to as micronutrients.

Although water, like oxygen from the air, is also essential for life, it is not usually considered as a food or a nutrient. The carbohydrate compounds, known collectively as 'fibre', are not strictly nutrients but have positive effects on our health. On the other hand, alcohol would be considered a food because it provides energy, even though it has drug-like properties. Iron from a cooking utensil (for example) is also a nutrient since it may be used to renew substances in the blood.

Hardly any foods contain only one nutrient. Most are very complex mixtures, which consist mainly of a variety of carbohydrates, fats and proteins, together with water. Minerals and vitamins are present in very much smaller amounts. One hundred grams (g) of potatoes, for example, contain about 18 g carbohydrates, 2 g proteins, 80 g water, some fibre and, if fried, they will also contain fat, but less than 50 mg in total of minerals and vitamins.

Energy

Energy is needed for the body to function and be active. The body derives energy from carbohydrates, fat, protein and alcohol in the diet. Experiments show that almost exactly the same amount of energy is produced from, say, wheat when it is eaten by humans as when it is used for fuel in a railway engine (as it has been in times of glut). The essential difference between the two chemical processes is that in the body the energy is released gradually by a series of steps, each carefully controlled by an enzyme.[2] This energy is used to perform muscular work and to maintain body temperature and such processes as breathing, but a considerable amount is also lost as heat. The energy provided by carbohydrate, fat, protein and other constituents can be measured and used to calculate the energy value of any food (see p. 32).

Other constituents of food

WATER

Water comprises about two-thirds of the body's weight, and is the medium or solvent in which almost every body process takes place both inside and outside the cells. The need of the body for water is second only to its need for air: adults

---

[1] *Vitamins* differ from hormones (which also help to regulate body processes) in that, with the exception of vitamin D, they cannot be made in the body and must therefore be supplied in the diet; hormones are always made within the body itself.

[2] *Enzymes* are special proteins, each of which accelerates the rate of a specific chemical reaction without itself being affected. They enable complex changes to occur in the body that would otherwise require more extreme conditions; without them life could not exist. To be active many require the presence of vitamins or minerals as 'co-factors'.

can survive for many weeks without food but for only a few days without water. Water is lost from the body in various ways. As the body works it produces waste products which could be toxic to the body and some are excreted through the kidneys in the urine. Water is also lost by evaporation in the breath and as sweat. Water is taken into the body from solid foods as well as from drinks (p. 33). The balance of water retained within the body is normally carefully regulated by the kidneys, but excessive losses can result from vomiting or diarrhoea in illness, or from heavy sweating due to strenuous activity or a hot climate. Then, if water intake is not increased, dehydration may result. In temperate climates such as that of the UK about 1.2 litres (6 to 8 glasses) of water or other fluids are required each day to maintain balance and prevent dehydration. However, this quantity should be increased when activity increases or the external temperature rises.

FIBRE

Some foods, particularly wholegrain cereals, pulses and some fruit and vegetables, contain substantial amounts of fibre (non-starch polysaccharides - see p. 7 and 11). Insoluble fibre fractions are not absorbed into the body; instead they add bulk to the faeces. This property is beneficial to health, in helping to prevent constipation. Soluble fibre constituents, which may be absorbed, are found especially in fruit, vegetables and pulses and can help to reduce the amount of cholesterol in the blood. However, fibre can also decrease the absorption of certain nutrients - especially some of the minerals. Fibre is further discussed on p. 7.

FLAVOURS AND COLOURS

In addition to the main nutritive and structural components, foods also contain innumerable minor constituents which give them their characteristic flavours, colours and textures. Control over the changes which occur in these constituents after ripening, and during storage, preparation and cooking, is an important consideration for both chefs and food technologists.

However, there is also increasing interest in this variety of biologically active compounds in relation to health. The compounds that colour foods such as carotenoids (yellow or orange pigments), anthocyanins (red and purple pigments), the flavonoids and other phenolic compounds found particularly in fruits, vegetables, tea and wine have antioxidant properties and increased consumption of some of these compounds is associated with a reduced risk of heart disease.

Malnutrition

The maintenance of health in an individual depends upon the consumption and absorption of appropriate amounts of energy and all the nutrients. Too little or too much of some, usually over a period of months or longer, may lead to ill health or malnutrition. Although the body has considerable power to adapt to reduced dietary intakes, for example by reduced physical activity, too low an intake of food will eventually result in *undernutrition* and, in extreme cases, *starvation*.

3

An example is the wasting (marasmus) in young children and stunting of physical and perhaps even mental development, which may result from inadequate breast feeding or from a poor weaning diet in developing countries. Other examples include the 'classical' nutrition deficiency diseases such as scurvy and some anaemias which result from diets containing too little of one or more vitamins or minerals, or from a physiological inability to absorb these nutrients. Excessive fatness (obesity), resulting from too great a food intake for the body's needs, is also a form of malnutrition, as is the excessive consumption of any nutrient, whether fat, sugar, mineral or vitamin, if it leads to ill health.

Units of measurement

Standard units are used to calculate the energy and nutrients in various amounts of food, and to measure heights and weights. The metric system (including the form known as SI[3]) has mainly been used in this edition of the manual. The relationships between these and traditional units are given in detail in Appendix 1.

---

[3] This system mainly affects the definition of energy, which has been measured in *kilocalories* (1 kcal being the amount of heat required to raise the temperature of 1 kg of water by 1°C). The SI unit, the *joule*, is hard to define in familiar terms, but 1 *kilojoule* (kJ) may be thought of as the amount of heat required to raise the temperature of 239 g of water by 1°C. 1 *megajoule* (1MJ) = 1000 kJ.

2 Carbohydrates

There are three major groups of carbohydrates in food: *sugars*, *starches* and *non-starch polysaccharides* (NSP). All are compounds of carbon, hydrogen and oxygen only, and their chemical structures are all based on a common unit (usually glucose). The units can be linked together in varying ways and in different numbers, and classification of the carbohydrates depends primarily on the number of units which varies from one to many thousands. Sugars and starches are a major source of food energy for humans throughout the world. Non-starch polysaccharides are known collectively as *fibre*.

Sugars

MONOSACCHARIDES (OR SIMPLE SUGARS)

Glucose (dextrose) occurs naturally in fruit and plant juices and in the blood of living animals. Most carbohydrates in food are ultimately converted to glucose during digestion. Glucose can also be manufactured from starch by the action of acid or specific enzymes. *Glucose syrups* (liquid glucose) result from the hydrolysis of starch (usually maize or wheat starch), and contain variable concentrations of glucose, maltose and various more complex carbohydrates depending on the end use for which they are intended. Except where the syrup is almost pure glucose, these syrups are less sweet than glucose. They are used in many manufactured foods including sugar confectionery, soft drinks and jams. Dried glucose is also made for domestic and industrial use.

Fructose occurs naturally in some fruit and vegetables and especially in honey. It is the sweetest sugar known. It is also a component of sucrose, from which it may be derived. The conversion of some of the glucose in glucose syrup to fructose results in the production of 'high fructose' syrups.

Galactose occurs mainly as part of lactose, but can be found as galactose in some foods.

DISACCHARIDES

Disaccharides consist of two monosaccharides linked together (minus the elements of water).

Sucrose occurs naturally in sugar cane and sugar beet, and in lesser amounts in fruits and some root vegetables such as carrots. It is a chemical combination of glucose and fructose. 'Sugar', whether white or brown, is essentially pure sucrose.

Maltose is formed during the breakdown of starch by digestion and, for example, when grain is germinated for the production of malt liquors such as beer. It is a combination of two glucose units.

Lactose occurs only in milk, including human milk. It is less sweet than sucrose or glucose, and is a combination of glucose and galactose. In its isolated form, it is added to some food products including meat products and some infant foods. Many individuals, particularly those of African, Asian and Indian races, have a limited ability to digest lactose. In later life some of these people may develop *lactose intolerance*, which results in digestive disturbances when the equivalent of a glass or more of milk is drunk. It is rarely found in healthy infants who depend on milk.

Properties of sugars

All sugars, whether monosaccharides or disaccharides, dissolve in water but vary in sweetness. Their taste may be modified by cooking (e.g. by caramelization). They usually form white (colourless) crystals when the water in which they are dissolved becomes supersaturated, but impure preparations may be brown. In addition to sweetness they provide a readily available source of energy; monosaccharides provide 16 kJ (3.75 kcal) per gram and disaccharides 17 kJ (4 kcal) per gram. Sugars can be used for several purposes in food preparation. For example, in jam-making and bottling they act as preservatives, and in biscuits, cakes, soft drinks and certain other foods, they also help to provide the characteristic texture and consistency.

Non-sugar sweeteners

Some other substances also taste sweet. *Sorbitol, mannitol* and *xylitol* are polyols (also known as sugar alcohols) which are made from sugars. Their energy value is similar to that of glucose, but for labelling purposes they are deemed to provide 10 kJ (2.4 kcal) per gram. In contrast, the intense sweeteners saccharin, aspartame and acesulfame K are classed as food additives as they have no chemical or nutritional relationship to sugars. They are about 200-500 times sweeter than sucrose and consequently used at a very low level so that even aspartame, which is the only one metabolised by the body, provides essentially no energy. They are used as sweetening agents to restrict the amount of sugars in the diet. Certain sweetening agents available in a granulated form (for example to sprinkle on breakfast cereals) are mixtures of an intense sweetener and a carbohydrate diluent and as such are sources of energy, although substantially less than the equivalent amount of sugar.

Starch

There are a number of starches, which are *polysaccharides* composed of variably large numbers of glucose units linked together to form both straight and branched chains (*amylose* and *amylopectin*, respectively). They exist in granules of a size and shape which are characteristic for each plant. In this form they are insoluble in water, and foods such as flour and potatoes, which contain large amounts of them, are indigestible if eaten raw. When heated or cooked in the presence of water, the starch granules swell and eventually gelatinise. They can then be more easily digested. One gram of starch provides approximately 17.6 kJ (4.2 kcal) of energy, but for food labelling purposes a value of 17 kJ (4 kcal) is used. Some forms of processing, for example dry heat used in the manufacture of certain breakfast cereals, can make part of the starch indigestible. Some scientists regard this fraction, known as *resistant starch*, as fibre along with non-starch polysaccharides (see below)

Glycogen is similar to starch in composition, but is made from glucose primarily by animals, including humans. Small amounts are stored in the liver and muscles as an energy reserve. It is not a significant item in the diet because it breaks down again to glucose after an animal's death.

Non-starch polysaccharides (NSP)

In addition to starch there are other polysaccharides found in the cell walls of vegetables, fruits, pulses and cereal grains where they provide part of the plant structure. This range of diverse compounds, when forming part of the human diet, is classified as *fibre* (Table 2). The non-starch polysaccharides in wheat, maize and rice are mainly insoluble cellulose and related materials, but those in fruits, vegetables and the cereals oats, barley and rye also contain soluble forms including pectins and gums.

Cellulose consists of many thousands of glucose units. It cannot be digested by humans, but can be used as food by cows and other ruminants whose digestive tract contains microorganisms capable of breaking it down into glucose. Cellulose and other indigestible polysaccharides add bulk to the faeces because of their water-binding capacity, and greatly assist the passage of digestible materials and waste products through the intestines, thus helping to prevent constipation.

Pectin is present in apples and many other fruits and in roots such as turnips and sweet potatoes. Its property of forming a stiff jelly is important in jam-making. Pectin is not fibrous, and because it is completely digested it has little effect on the faeces. However, pectin and other soluble fibre components can help to reduce the amount of cholesterol in the blood.

As the effects of both soluble and insoluble NSP are beneficial, it is best to include a variety of NSP-rich foods in the diet. National dietary guidelines recommend consumption of a naturally high fibre diet. Daily intakes of NSP in the UK average 15.2 g for men and significantly lower, 12.6 g, for women, being provided mainly by vegetables and cereals. About a third of men and half of women have intakes below 12 g per day. It has been recommended, however, that population average intakes of NSP should rise to 18 g per day (see p. 81).

Fibre components can bind minerals such as calcium, iron, copper and zinc making them unavailable to the body. However, the only people likely to be adversely affected by high-fibre diets are those who have a low or marginal mineral intake.

Sources of carbohydrates in the diet

Plants form sugars in their leaves by the action of sunlight, but store them in their stems, roots, tubers or seeds as starch (the small amount of starch stored in unripe fruits, however, turns back into glucose or sucrose on ripening). Starch forms the major energy reserve of most plants, and thus in turn provides a major part of food energy for humans. The principal sources of sugars in the diet are milk (lactose), fruit and honey (fructose), sucrose, glucose syrups and fruit juices used both alone and in jams, canned fruit, cakes, biscuits, ice cream and other foods prepared in the home or by food manufacturers.

The sugars and starch contents of selected foods are shown in Table 1. Twenty seven per cent of the present intake of carbohydrate in the UK consists of sucrose and glucose syrups, 16 per cent is lactose and the sugars which occur naturally in foods such as whole fruits, and the remainder, starch. A century ago, flour and potato consumption was much higher and sucrose consumption much lower. Then, as in the developing countries now, starch was a much more important component of the diet. By 2001, however, the proportions of dietary energy provided by total sugars and starch were more similar (23 and 30 per cent, respectively). The main food sources of carbohydrates are shown at the foot of Table 1. The total fibre content of the average UK diet has not changed much over the past century, but a greater proportion now comes from vegetables and less from cereals as a result of changing eating habits. There has, however, been an increase in recent years in the consumption of whole meal bread and bran-containing breakfast cereals.

Table 1. Average carbohydrate content of selected foods (edible portion)

	Available carbohydrate, as monosaccharides		
	Sugars (g/100 g)	Starch (g/100 g)	Total (g/100 g)
Whole milk[a]	4.5	0.0	4.5
Skimmed milk[a]	4.4	0.0	4.4
Ice cream (non-dairy)	18.8	0.0	18.8
Meat	0.0	0.0	0.0
Sugar[b]	105.0	0.0	105.0
Honey	76.4	0.0	76.4
Jam	69.0	0.0	69.0
Baked beans	5.9	9.4	15.3
Potatoes, old, boiled	0.7	16.3	17.0
Macaroni, boiled	0.3	18.2	18.5
Rice, white, boiled	0.0	30.9	30.9
Bananas	20.9	2.3	23.2
Oranges	8.5	0.0	8.5
Peaches canned in syrup	14.0	0.0	14.0
Peaches canned in juice	9.7	0.0	9.7
Sultanas	69.4	0.0	69.4
Biscuits, chocolate, fully coated	45.8	21.8	67.6
Bread, white	3.4	42.7	46.1
Bread, wholemeal	2.8	39.3	42.0
Flour, white, plain	1.5	76.2	77.7
Cornflakes	8.2	81.4	89.6
Muesli, Swiss style (with added sugar)	26.2	46.0	72.2
Muesli, no added sugar	15.7	51.4	67.1
Porridge, made with water	0.1	8.0	8.1
Orange juice, unsweetened	8.8	0.0	8.8
Cola	10.9	0.0	10.9
Soup, canned, cream of tomato	2.6	3.3	5.9
Tomato ketchup	27.5	1.1	28.6
Milk chocolate	56.9	0.0	56.9
Plain chocolate	62.6	0.0	62.6
Lager	0.0	0.0	0.0
Wine, white, medium	3.0	0.0	3.0

[a] Lactose
[b] Equivalent to 100 g of sucrose

1g of disaccharide is equivalent to 1.05 g of monosaccharide.

1g of starch is equivalent to 1.10 g of monosaccharide.

The main sources of sugars in the diet are table sugar, soft drinks, biscuits, cake and pastries, chocolate, beer and lager, fruit and fruit juice, milk (as lactose) and bread. The main sources of starches in the diet are cereals and cereal products (especially bread and breakfast cereals), and potatoes.

Health aspects of carbohydrates

Although all sugars and starches absorbed by the body provide similar amounts of energy, they have different physiological effects. Eating a lot of certain types of sugary foods at frequent intervals, especially between meals, is associated with increased tooth decay (dental caries). In a 1989 report, the Government's advisory Committee on Medical Aspects of Food and Nutrition Policy (COMA)[1] considered that the type of sugars and its location within a food can affect its ability to cause dental caries, and that it is useful to classify sugars in the following way:

Intrinsic sugars are those contained within the cell walls of food, e.g. sugars in whole fruits and vegetables.

Extrinsic sugars are those not contained within the cell structure of a food and include:

Milk sugars, which occur naturally in milk and milk products (almost all lactose).

Non-milk extrinsic (NME) sugars, e.g. sugars in fruit juices, table sugar, sugars added to food including honey, glucose syrups, maple syrup etc.

Intrinsic and milk sugars are not considered to have adverse effects on teeth. NME sugars, on the other hand, can play a significant part in tooth decay, although regular brushing of teeth and the use of fluoride toothpaste can lessen this effect.

When it is desirable to reduce the fat content of the diet, a good way of replacing the lost energy is by increasing the intake of fibre-rich starchy foods. NME sugars should contribute no more than 10 per cent of dietary energy on average for the population. In 2001, both men and women were consuming more than the recommended level of NME sugars at an average of 13.6 and 11.9 per cent of food energy, respectively. In the same year, the mean percentage food energy derived from starch and intrinsic and milk sugars for the population was below the recommended 39 per cent.

The target for NSP has already been mentioned (see p. 7). Because of these targets, it is useful to know the amounts of different types of carbohydrate in foods. Examples are shown in Tables 1 and 2.

---

[1] COMA was replaced in 2000 by the Scientific Advisory Committee on Nutrition (SACN), which advises the UK Health Departments, and the Food Standards Agency on scientific aspects of nutrition and health.

Table 2. Fibre content of selected foods (edible portion), expressed as non-starch polysaccharide and total dietary fibre (AOAC)

	Non-starch polysaccharides (g/100 g)	Total dietary fibre (AOAC) (g/100 g)
Meat	0.0	0.0
Low fat yogurt, fruit	0.2	0.3
Baked beans	3.7	n/a
Beans, red kidney, boiled	6.7	n/a
Beans, runner, boiled	1.9	n/a
Broccoli, boiled	2.3	n/a
Carrots, boiled	2.5	n/a
Potatoes, cooked	1.9	2.4
Tomatoes, raw	1.0	n/a
Apples with skin, eating	1.8	n/a
Bananas	1.1	n/a
Mixed nuts	6.0	n/a
Scones, fruit	2.0	2.9
Biscuits, semi-sweet, e.g. rich tea	1.7	n/a
Bread, white	1.9	2.5
Bread, brown	3.5	5.0
Bread, wholemeal	5.0	7.0
Wheat flour, white	3.1	n/a
Wheat flour, brown	6.4	n/a
Wheat flour, wholemeal	9.0	n/a
Bran type cereal e.g. All Bran	24.5	n/a
Oatmeal	7.1	n/a
Toasted rice cereal e.g. Rice Krispies	0.7	n/a
Shredded wheat type cereal	9.8	n/a
Wheat biscuits e.g. Weetabix	9.7	n/a
Rice, egg fried, takeaway	0.8	1.1
Rice, brown, boiled	0.8	n/a
Dried spaghetti, white, boiled	1.5	1.7
Dried spaghetti, wholewheat, boiled	4.4	4.2

The main sources of fibre in the diet are bread and other cereal products, vegetables and fruit.

Table 2 shows two fibre values for some selected foods. One value is fibre determined as NSP by the Englyst method, which has traditionally been used in the UK and Ireland; the other is fibre determined as NSP plus resistant starch and lignin by the Association of Analytical Chemists (AOAC) method used in other European countries. In general the AOAC method tends to give higher values than Englyst, the magnitude of the difference varying between foods, which makes it difficult to compare fibre contents of foods produced in different countries. The Government has recommended that AOAC values be used for nutrition labelling purposes in the UK.

Diabetes is discussed on pp. 29 and 132.

3   Fats

Fats include not only 'visible fats' such as butter and margarine, cooking fats and oils and the fat on meat, but also the 'invisible fats' which occur in foods such as cheese, biscuits and cakes, nuts and other foods of animal and vegetable origin. They are a more concentrated source of energy than carbohydrates, and are the form in which much of the energy reserve of animals and some seeds is stored.

Like carbohydrates, fats are compounds of carbon, hydrogen and oxygen only, but the proportion of oxygen is lower. Chemically, fats in food consist mainly of mixtures of *triglycerides*. Each triglyceride is a combination of three *fatty acids* with a unit of glycerol (glycerine), and the differences between one fat or oil and another are largely the result of the different fatty acids in each.

Fatty acids

Many different fatty acids are found in nature. They differ in the number of carbon atoms they contain, and the number of hydrogen atoms held by the carbon atoms. *Saturated* fatty acids have as many hydrogen atoms as they can hold and this makes them stable so that they keep well. When hydrogen atoms are missing, carbon atoms form double bonds. *Monounsaturated* fatty acids contain only one double bond (two missing hydrogen atoms). *Polyunsaturated* fatty acids have two or more double bonds (four or more missing hydrogen atoms) which react gradually with oxygen in the air and make the fat rancid. All fats contain a mixture of these three types of fatty acid, but in widely varying proportions, depending on the source (Table 3 and Appendix 3). The presence of large amounts of unsaturated fatty acids in a mixture affects the physical as well as the chemical properties of a fat, making it liquid at room temperature (i.e. an oil). Fats that are solid at room temperature for example beef fat, contain most of their fatty acids as saturates and monounsaturates. Some vegetable oils such as coconut and palm oils have a relatively high proportion of saturated fatty acids, but because these have a relatively low number of carbon atoms they do not cause the oil to solidify. In nature unsaturated fatty acids generally have their double bonds in the *cis* form. They can be changed into saturated fatty acids and a mixture of *cis* and *trans* monounsaturated fatty acids by controlled treatment with hydrogen (hydrogenation). This happens when liquid oils are hardened in the manufacture of margarine, fat spreads and cooking fats and, to a lesser extent, in the rumen of cows and sheep. The more important fatty acids in foods are as follows:

SATURATED FATTY ACIDS

Palmitic acid and *stearic acid* are major constituents of hard fats such as butter, lard, suet and cocoa butter. *Myristic acid* occurs in butter and coconut oil.

Butyric acid, which, although present in only small amounts in milk fat and butter, makes an important contribution to their taste. Free butyric acid is released when these fats become rancid.

Table 3. Average fatty acid composition of some foods

	Fat (g/100g edible portion)	Fatty acids[a] (g/100g edible portion)			
		Saturated	Mono-unsaturated	Poly-unsaturated	Trans
Milk, cow's, semi-skimmed	1.7	1.1	0.4	0.0	0.1
Milk, human	4.1	1.8	1.6	0.5	N
Cheese, Cheddar	34.9	21.7	9.4	1.1	1.4
Eggs, chicken, raw	11.2	3.2	4.4	1.7	0.1
Beef, mince, raw	16.2[b]	6.9	6.9	0.5	0.8
Pork, chops, lean and fat, raw	21.7	8.0	8.5	3.6	0.1
Chicken, meat average, raw	2.1	0.6	1.0	0.4	0.0
Liver, lamb, raw	6.2	1.7	1.8	0.9	0.0
Sardines, canned in tomato sauce	9.9	2.8	2.9	3.2	0.0
Butter	82.2	52.1	20.9	2.8	2.9
Margarine, hard	79.3	34.6	36.2	5.4	12.2
Margarine, soft	81.7	27.2	38.9	12.4	8.9
Margarine, polyunsaturated	82.8	17.0	26.6	36.0	6.7
Sunflower oil	99.9	12.0	20.5	63.3	0.0
Olive oil	99.9	14.3	73.0	8.2	0.0
Blended vegetable oil[c]	99.9	11.7	53.2	29.8	0.0
Potato crisps	34.2	14.0	13.7	5.0	N
Peanuts, dry roasted	49.8	8.9	22.8	15.5	0.0
Chocolate chip cookies	22.9	10.6	8.6	2.6	0.3
Chocolate, milk	30.7	18.3	9.9	1.2	0.4

[a] The fatty acids add up to less than the total fat because fat also contains glycerol, phospholipids, sterols and other fatty compounds.
[b] Average of values that ranged from 7.8g to 26.5g per 100g
[c] Average of several kinds; fatty acid profile of any one kind will depend on the particular blend of oils used in its manufacture.
N - The nutrient is present in significant quantities but there is no reliable information on the amount

UNSATURATED FATTY ACIDS

Monounsaturates
Oleic acid occurs in substantial amounts in all fats, but especially in olive oil and rapeseed (canola) oil where it provides 60-70 per cent of the total fatty acid content. *Trans* isomers of oleic and other monounsaturated fatty acids are found in hard margarines and shortenings and in products made from them such as biscuits and pastries, and in lesser amounts in soft margarines and reduced fat spreads and ruminant fats (milk, cheese, beef and lamb).

Polyunsaturates
Linoleic acid (with two double bonds) occurs in large amounts in vegetable seed oils such as maize (corn), soya bean and sunflower seed oils, and in small amounts in some animal fats such as pork.
Alpha-linolenic acid (with three double bonds) occurs in small amounts in vegetable oils.
Arachidonic acid (with four double bonds) occurs in very small amounts in some animal fats. It can be formed in the body from linoleic acid.

A number of other polyunsaturated fatty acids occur in plants and fish oils, and are thought to be particularly beneficial to health. They include *gamma linolenic acid* (GLA), and the long chain polyunsaturated fatty acids (LCPUFAs) *eicosapentaenoic acid* (EPA) and *docosahexaenoic acid* (DHA).

Polyunsaturated fatty acids can also be classified into *omega-3* (n-3) or *omega-6* (n-6) families, according to the position of the double bonds. Both *omega-3* and *omega-6* polyunsaturated fatty acids must be present in the diet for normal health. Linoleic and alpha-linolenic acids are called 'essential fatty acids' because they cannot be made in the body. Arachidonic acid is sometimes regarded as essential if alpha-linolenic acid is in short supply. It is therefore unwise to aim for a fat-free diet in the mistaken idea that this is a 'healthy diet'. These fatty acids are required in small quantities in the diet for metabolism in the body to two families of *omega-3* and *omega-6* fatty acids, which are necessary for the structure and functions of the tissues.

Alpha-linolenic acid is the starting point for the production, in the body, of EPA, which in turn gives rise to DHA through a series of chemical reactions catalysed by various enzymes which lengthen and desaturate the fatty acid chains. DHA and EPA, which are obtained in the diet principally from oily fish, and alpha-linolenic acid all belong to the *omega-3* family. Some *omega-3* fatty acids are found in certain vegetable oils such as linseed, flaxseed, walnut and rapeseed oils, but are not the same type of fatty acids nor do they have the same beneficial effects as those found in oily fish.

Linoleic, GLA and arachidonic acids in turn are transformed in the body to longer chain fatty acids which belong to the *omega-6* family. They are also obtained in the diet mainly from vegetable seeds and polyunsaturated margarines.

Properties of fats

Fats are solid at low temperatures and become liquid when they are heated. Oils are simply fats which are liquid at room temperature, usually as a result of their higher content of unsaturated fatty acids, and solidify on refrigeration (e.g. olive oil). Oils and fats do not dissolve in water, but may be *emulsified* with water by vigorous mixing as when butter, margarine and reduced-fat spreads are made. The oil and water usually separate again unless emulsifiers such as lecithin from soya beans or egg are added to the mixture.

Fats make an important contribution to food characteristics such as texture and palatability. Food fats usually contain small amounts of other fat-soluble substances, including flavour components and some of the vitamins. Animal fats may contain retinol (vitamin A) and vitamin D, and varying amounts of cholesterol, while vegetable fats may contain carotenes (which can be converted into vitamin A in the body) and vitamin E, but do not contain cholesterol.

The amount of energy obtained from a given weight of all common fats is about the same, despite the different functions and properties of many of the component fatty acids. It is more than double the energy, at 37 kJ per gram (9 kcal per gram), of an equal weight of carbohydrate or protein (see p. 32).

Mineral oils, such as liquid paraffin, are chemically different from food fats and oils despite their similarity in appearance. They cannot be utilised by the body, but function as laxatives and will reduce the absorption of some nutrients.

Sources of fat in the diet

VEGETABLE SOURCES

In plants, fats are formed from carbohydrate. Thus, when seeds such as sunflower and cottonseed ripen, their starch content decreases as their fat content rises. Oilseeds such as these and peanuts, coconuts, rapeseeds, palm kernels and soya beans contain about 20-40 per cent oil and are among the chief sources of oil for the manufacture of margarine and cooking fat. The fat content of flour and other cereal products (apart from oatmeal) is generally low, as is the fat content of most vegetables and fruits. The proportion of each fatty acid present varies from plant to plant, and is also quite variable within a species. Vegetable seeds are among the principal sources of *omega-6* polyunsaturated fatty acids.

ANIMAL SOURCES

Animals, including humans, store excess energy almost entirely in deposits of fat, the amount of which is very variable. As in plants, this fat can be made from carbohydrate, but the dietary carbohydrate can be starch, sugar or even (in cows and sheep) cellulose. Animals also lay down fat from their dietary fat; in this case the fatty acid composition reflects that of the diet, except for ruminants whose digestive processes normally make the fatty acids more saturated.

Fish such as herring, mackerel, pilchards, salmon, sardines, tuna and eels are sometimes called *oily fish*. The proportion of fat in them varies with the season of the year. Fish oils are the principal sources of *omega-3* polyunsaturated fatty acids, including the long chain polyunsaturated fatty acids. *White fish* such as cod, haddock and plaice contain little fat except in the liver. Fish liver is also a rich source of vitamins A and D.

The fat content of many foods, especially meat, varies widely. Average values, and the main sources of fat in the British diet, are shown in Table 4.

Table 4. Average fat content of foods, uncooked[a] (edible portion)

	Fat (g/100 g)		Fat (g/100 g)
Milk, whole	3.9	Cod, filleted	0. 7
Milk, semi-skimmed	1.7	Mackerel	16.1[b]
Milk, skimmed	0.2	Tuna, canned in oil, drained	9.0
Cream, double	53.7	Tuna, canned in brine	0.6
Yogurt, low fat, fruit	1.1	Butter	82.2
Ice cream, non-dairy	7.8	Margarine, soft, poly unsaturated	82.8
Cheese, Cheddar	34.9	Fat spread, 40% fat	37.5
Cheese, Edam	26.0	Fat spread, 20-25% fat	25.5
Cheese, cottage, plain	4.3	Vegetable oils	99.9
Eggs	11.2	Lard and dripping	99.0
Beef, stewing steak	6.4	Ghee, vegetable	99.4
Lamb, leg, lean and fat	12.3	Potatoes, old	0.2
Pork, chop, lean and fat	21.7	Chips, takeaway	12.4[c]
Bacon, streaky	23.6	Chips, oven-baked	4.2
Sausages, pork	25.0	Peanut butter, smooth	51.8
Ham	3.3	Bread, white	1.6
Beefburgers	24.7	Bread, wholemeal	2.5
Chicken, dark and light meat	2.1	Porridge oats	7.8
Turkey, dark and light meat	1.6	Biscuits, digestive, plain	20.3

The main sources of fat in the diet are meat and meat products, cereals and cereal products (including biscuits, buns, cakes and pastries), milk and milk products, fat spreads, potato chips and savoury snacks.
[a] Unless otherwise stated.
[b] Levels range from 6 to 23g fat per 100g.
[c] Content variable and depends on a number of factors relating to preparation.

Throughout the world the amount of fat in the diet tends to be higher in affluent than in poor countries, and within poorer countries, higher in the wealthier families. Less than 10 per cent of the energy value of the diet is derived from fat in many of the world's poorest countries. In most developed countries, including Britain, fat provided about 40 per cent of energy for many years, but in Britain this proportion has fallen to about 35 per cent in recent years.

The amount of dietary energy derived from saturated fatty acids has been falling and the average proportion of polyunsaturated to saturated fatty acids (the 'P/S ratio') in the whole diet is about 0.5:1, having risen from about 0.2:1 in 1970.

Health aspects of fats

Diets in poor countries are often low in energy, and the World Health Organization (WHO) has recommended an increase in fat intakes in such situations. More affluent populations need to moderate their fat intake to prevent an excess of energy intake over expenditure leading to weight gain, and particularly to decrease the saturated fatty acid content of their diets as a means of reducing the risk of heart disease.

To ensure that sufficient quantities of essential fatty acids are present in our diets, it is recommended that linoleic and alpha-linolenic acids (which were once called vitamin F), should provide at least I and 0.2 per cent, respectively, of the total dietary energy. At the same time, to encourage a decrease in total fat and saturated fatty acid intake, there is a set of average values that are advisable for the UK population to achieve in terms of the proportion of dietary energy to be consumed as different types of fatty acids (see overleaf).

HEART DISEASE

In the UK, in both men and women, *coronary heart disease* (CHD) is a serious health problem. The risk of heart disease is increased by various factors such as smoking, high blood pressure and raised levels of cholesterol in the blood. All, except smoking, are influenced by the diet. Obesity can affect both blood pressure and blood cholesterol and is discussed on p. 29. Blood pressure can also be increased by excessive intakes of alcohol (see p. 112) and by obesity. It may also be raised by high intakes of sodium. High saturated fatty acid intakes can lead to increased blood cholesterol levels, particularly in susceptible individuals.

Cholesterol is mostly made in the liver and is carried in the blood mainly by two proteins - *low-density lipoprotein* (LDL) and *high-density lipoprotein* (HDL). LDL cholesterol is considered to be undesirable because if it increases to a high level in the blood it can be deposited on the walls of the blood vessels thereby helping to form 'plaques' that may eventually lead to narrowing of the arteries that supply the heart with blood. This is more likely to happen if the LDL is modified chemically by oxidation (p. 75). If the arteries become blocked completely with further plaque or by a blood clot, the blood supply to the heart is interrupted leading to a heart attack and, in severe cases, to death. HDL cholesterol is desirable as it is a means of transporting cholesterol, from parts of the body where there is too much, to the liver where it is disposed. Replacing saturated by monunsaturated or polyunsaturated fatty acids in the diet can lower LDL blood cholesterol. The cholesterol in food has a smaller effect on blood cholesterol than do saturated fatty acids, but the effect varies in different people. The liver can compensate for changes in dietary cholesterol by changing the amount of cholesterol it makes.

The long chain *omega*-3 polyunsaturated fatty acids in fish oils do not seem to have a major effect on blood cholesterol levels, but may help to prevent heart disease by decreasing the tendency of the blood to clot and keeping the heart cell membranes stable. Current recommendations are that the average intake of long chain *omega*-3 polyunsaturated fatty acids for the population should double to about 0.2 g per day (1.5 g per week). This would be achieved by increasing consumption of oily fish. Recent evidence suggests that the *omega*-3 polyunsaturates found in vegetable sources (see **Unsaturated fatty acids** p. 14) may not have the same beneficial effects as those found in oily fish.

In order to help achieve a decrease in heart disease the Government advises that: on average, total fat and saturated fatty acids should provide not more than about 35 per cent and 10 per cent, respectively, of dietary energy intake; omega-6 polyunsaturated fatty acids should continue to provide about 6 per cent of energy; and the average intake of dietary cholesterol should not increase. Between 1986 and 2001, fat and saturated fatty acid contributions to food energy intake fell from about 43 to 35 per cent and from about 18 to 13 per cent, respectively. In spite of these encouraging trends the top 2.5% of people surveyed in 2000 - 01 were getting almost 50% of their energy from fat. Many people therefore still need to be encouraged to make substantial changes to their diets if the average population intake of saturated fatty acids, is to decrease to the desired level.

Trans unsaturated fatty acids

Fats containing *trans* unsaturated fatty acids (*trans* fats) occur in nature in dairy produce and the flesh of ruminants, e.g. beef, lamb. Partially hydrogenated vegetable oils also contain *trans* fats, which are produced during the process of hydrogenation used to turn liquid oil into solid fat; this is the main source of *trans* fats in the UK diet.

Trans fats have been shown to raise blood cholesterol levels and increase the risk of coronary heart disease. The adverse effect of *trans* fatty acids is similar to that of saturated fatty acids (found in animal fats and dairy produce). However, the quantity of *trans* fats from partially hydrogenated vegetable oils in the average diet is much lower than that of saturated fats, and average dietary intake has been reduced since partially hydrogenated vegetable oils were removed from UK margarines.

Current average dietary intakes are lower than the 1994 COMA[1] recommendation of about 2.0% total energy, or 5g per day. In 1986/87 average intakes were 2.0% of total energy and by 2000/01 this had reduced to an average intake of 1.1% of total energy).

---

[1] COMA was replaced in 2000 by SACN– see p. 10.

CANCER

In a report published in 1998, COMA[1] concluded that there was not sufficiently strong evidence linking total fat intakes to the development of cancers to make any specific recommendations. The report's recommendations include maintenance of a healthy body weight and increased intakes of a variety of fruit and vegetables and of fibre from a variety of food sources. For adults, it also recommends that individuals' intake of red and processed meat should not increase and that high consumers of these foods should consider a reduction. As a guide, average UK intakes are about 90 g per day and high intakes above 140 g per day (both on a cooked weight basis). These recommendations were made in the light of existing recommendations, including those to reduce the average fat intake of the population (see page 18).

4   Proteins

All proteins are compounds of carbon, hydrogen and oxygen, but unlike carbohydrates and fats, they always contain nitrogen as well. Most proteins also contain sulphur (present in only a few amino acids) and some contain phosphorus. They are essential constituents of all cells, where they regulate the processes of life or provide structure. Protein must be provided in the diet for the growth and repair of the body, but any excess is used to provide energy.

Proteins consist of chains of hundreds or even thousands of *amino acid* units. Only about 20 different amino acids are used, but the number of ways in which they can be arranged is almost infinite. It is the specific and unique sequence of these units that gives each protein its characteristic structural and enzymatic properties.

Amino acids

It is convenient to divide amino acids into two types: *indispensable* and *dispensable*. *Indispensable* amino acids cannot be made in the body, at least in amounts sufficient for health, and must therefore be present in the food. *Dispensable* amino acids are equally necessary as components of all proteins in the body; they differ only in that it is possible for them to be made from any excess of certain other amino acids in the diet. The eight amino acids indispensable for *adults* are:

Isoleucine	Phenylalanine
Leucine	Threonine
Lysine	Tryptophan
Methionine	Valine

A further amino acid, histidine, is also indispensable for the rapidly growing *infant*. The remaining amino acids which are found in proteins are:

Alanine	Glutamine
Arginine	Glycine
Aspartic acid	Proline
Asparagine	Serine
Cysteine	Tyrosine
Glutamic acid	

Animal and vegetable proteins

The overall proportions of amino acids in any single vegetable food (cereals, nuts and seeds, potatoes, or legumes such as peas and beans) differ from those needed by humans. For example, wheat and rice proteins are comparatively low in lysine, and legumes such as lentils are low in tryptophan and methionine (Table 5). These proteins are therefore said to have low *biological values*, because the *quality* of a protein depends on its ability to supply all the indispensable amino acids in the amounts needed. Mixtures of such foods, however, complement each other and result in greatly enhanced values so that, even among those who eat little or no animal protein, deficiency is rarely a problem provided they have enough food to eat.

Most animal proteins (from meat, fish, milk, cheese and eggs) have a high biological value. The reason for this is that humans are part of the animal kingdom; the proteins of animals are therefore more like ours and can be utilised by us with the minimum of waste. In effect, animals have pre-selected, with varying degrees of efficiency, the plant amino acids which they and we need and have burned up the remainder for energy (p. 40). Nevertheless, the nutritional advantages of foods of animal origin over those of vegetable origin lie, in practice,

Table 5. Proportion of some indispensable amino acids in selected proteins.

	Lysine	Methionine	Tryptophan
Milk, cow's	8.4	2.9	1.5
Eggs	6.2	3.1	1.8
Beef	9.1	2.7	1.3
Fish, cod	9.8	2.9	1.1
Lentils	6.7	0.7	0.9
Peanuts	4.0	1.3	1.3
Wheat flour[a]	2.7	1.8	1.3
Rice[a]	3.3	1.8	1.2

[a] Some amino acids can be increased by genetic breeding.

more in the presence of associated nutrients such as vitamin B_{12}, iron and retinol (pre-formed vitamin A) than in the protein.

Because there is no way in which excesses of amino acids can be stored in the body, they will be most efficiently used if a complete assortment is supplied to the body at about the same time. This can be achieved by eating a mixed diet at each meal and ensuring that the total energy content of the diet is also adequate. Mixtures of vegetable protein foods such as beans on toast, or of animal and vegetable foods such as fish and chips, bread and cheese, and breakfast cereals with milk, therefore have a sound physiological basis.

Novel sources of protein

Animals convert plant protein into their own muscle slowly and inefficiently (only 5-10 per cent being retained). Over recent years there has been a growing demand for sources of protein which are suitable for vegetarians. Some people may also want to limit their fat intake and eat protein-rich foods which are lower in fat.

As a response to these factors, products providing alternatives to meat have been developed by the food industry. In addition to those described below, soya-based foods such as tofu (bean curd) and miso (fermented bean paste), which are traditionally used in Far Eastern cuisine, are now increasingly available in the UK.

Texturised vegetable proteins have been developed by concentrating or isolating the proteins from a number of plants, especially soya beans, and converting them directly into products such as soya 'mince' or soya 'chunks'. If suitably fortified with the most important minerals and vitamins which meat provides, such as thiamin, riboflavin, vitamin B_{12}, iron and zinc, these products can be used instead of meat and are acceptable to vegetarians (vegetarian diets are discussed on p. 131).

Mycoprotein is another product which can be used as an alternative to meat. One type, made from a particular fungal microorganism and complying with a particular specification, has been cleared for human consumption. It is manufactured commercially (Quorn®) and is produced by growing the fungal microorganism in a fermenter and 'harvesting' the product. This is heat-processed, seasoned and cooked, and then sliced, diced or shredded. It can be used instead of meat in home recipes and is also incorporated into a range of retailed products, for example pies and recipe dishes.

It is also possible to utilise other microorganisms such as yeast, or otherwise inedible leaves, to provide protein-rich foods. Given that such foodstuffs would have a novel composition they would be subject to a stringent pre-market safety assessment.

Protein as a source of energy

The amount and type of protein in the diet will not exactly balance the requirements for growth, repair and maintenance: there will always be excesses of some amino acids, and usually an excess of total protein. These will be converted into glucose in the liver or be directly oxidised to provide heat and energy. Furthermore, if the energy available from the diet is insufficient to meet demands, this oxidation of the amino acids tends to take preference over their more fundamental use for rebuilding proteins. This is why it is important to ensure that diets contain sufficient energy in the form of carbohydrate and fat before proteins are added, for only then can these proteins be properly utilised for purposes which no other nutrient can fulfil.

Other health aspects of proteins

Newborn infants can absorb some proteins intact from their mothers' milk, including antibodies which provide protection from infection. Susceptible individuals can also react adversely to certain food proteins known as allergens: for example, those with coeliac disease react to gluten and others may react to cow's milk protein and nut proteins. Most allergic reactions to food are mild, but if someone has a food allergy they can react to tiny amounts of the food they are sensitive to, with fatal results in rare cases.

Certain beans, including red kidney beans and soya beans, contain proteins, which are harmful unless thoroughly cooked in *moist* heat such as boiling water.

Properties of proteins

Some proteins dissolve in water and some in salt water. Some are insoluble and this is exploited in the preparation of wheat gluten, which is used to improve the baking quality of wheats produced in the UK, by washing other proteins and starch from a wheat dough. The separated starch is used for producing glucose syrups.

The action of heat on proteins is complex. Proteins such as the albumen in egg white harden or coagulate irreversibly when heated, but are still readily digested. Individual amino acids are little affected by normal cooking procedures, although some of the lysine may react with carbohydrates in the food (e.g. in the baking of bread) and methionine may sometimes be reduced. In the preparation of gelatin, however, when connective tissue from meat is boiled for many hours, all the tryptophan is destroyed.

The complex Maillard reactions between amino acids (usually lysine) and sugars in foods result in the attractive golden brown colour of crisps or chips and also in the formation of certain desirable food flavours. However, they may also give rise to the brown discoloration which sometimes develops during prolonged storage of concentrated or dried milk or dehydrated vegetables.

Sources of protein in the diet

About one-third of the protein in the average UK diet comes from plant sources and two-thirds from animal sources. The amount of protein in nuts and dried peas and beans is very high - about the same as in meat, fish and cheese. The proportion is reduced when these pulses are soaked in water, but they remain an excellent source of protein. Cereals are also rich in protein; indeed wheat, maize and rice are the main sources of protein for many people in the world. The amount of protein in roots and tubers is small, but as potatoes are eaten in quantity they provide useful amounts. Many green and leafy vegetables contain some protein, but because they are often eaten in small amounts or infrequently by some sectors of the UK population they make little contribution to average protein intakes. The concentration of protein in selected foods is shown in Table 6.

Table 6. Average protein content of selected foods, uncooked[a]

	Protein (g/100 g)		Protein (g/100 g)
Milk, cow's, whole	3.3	Beans, red kidney, dry	22.1
Milk, cow's, skimmed	3.4	Soya tofu, steamed	8.1
Soya non-dairy alternative		Quorn (Mycoprotein)	16.1
to milk, unsweetened	2.4	Peanuts, plain	25.6
Cheese, Cheddar	25.4	Peas	6.9
Cheese, feta	15.6	Sweetcorn, canned	2.9
Beef, stewing, lean and fat	22.1	Potatoes, old	2.1
Lamb, leg, lean and fat	19.0	Apples, eating	0.4
Pork, chop, lean and fat	18.6	Bread, white	7.9
Sausages, pork	11.9	Bread, wholemeal	9.4
Chicken, dark and light meat	22.3	Flour, white	9.4
Turkey, dark and light meat	22.6	Cornflakes	7.9
Cod, fillets	18.3	Oatmeal	11.2
Prawns	17.6	Spaghetti, white, dry	12.0
Baked beans, reheated	5.2	Rice, white	7.4

The main sources of protein in the diet are meat and meat products, cereals and cereal products (especially bread), and milk and milk products.

[a] Unless otherwise stated

5 Energy needs and food consumption

Uses of energy

Energy, which gives us the ability to do work, is obtained from food by controlled oxidation of the carbohydrates, fat, protein and alcohol in the diet. It is necessary for three purposes:

(a) to maintain life
(b) for muscular activity, and
(c) for additional needs during growth, pregnancy and lactation.

If more is obtained than is used in these ways, the excess is stored in the body as fat.

MAINTENANCE OF LIFE

Energy is required for breathing, the heartbeat, the maintenance of body temperature, and other involuntary activities including brain function. The amount needed can be measured in people at complete rest. This *basal metabolic rate* (BMR) is higher in relation to body size in infants and actively growing young children than in adults. After adolescence, the needs are proportional to the amount of lean tissue in the body; thus women tend to have lower resting metabolic rates than men both because they are lighter and because muscle generally forms a lower proportion of their body weight (and fat a higher proportion). The BMR is also lower in elderly people, or during starvation, because of the reduction that occurs in lean tissue. It is thus possible to adapt to changed energy intakes.

After food is eaten, extra heat is produced and more energy is needed to cover this. The amount varies with the food. Climate does not significantly affect the resting metabolism, but the rate does vary widely between apparently similar individuals because the efficiency of the body processes varies. Average values of the BMR for the two sexes in different age groups can be estimated from body weight using the equations shown in Appendix 2.

Some examples are:

	Weight (kg)	Basal metabolic rate (BMR) (resting energy requirement)	
		MJ(kcal)/day	MJ (kcal)/kg/day
Infant, 1 year old	10	2.3 (560)	0.23 (56)
Boy, 10 years old	33	5.2 (1240)	0.16 (38)
Man, 40 years old	76	7.3 (1750)	0.10 (23)
Woman, 40 years old	62	5.7 (1360)	0.09 (22)
Man, 75+ years old	69	5.8 (1400)	0.08 (20)

A man therefore needs about 5 kJ (a little more than 1 kcal) each minute just to keep alive. During 8 hours sleep, the resting requirement of about 2.4 MJ (580 kcal) is all that would be used, but during the remainder of the day the additional requirements of physical activity must be taken into account.

ACTIVITY

Whenever people move, they use extra energy. The heavier they are the more it takes, and strenuous activities require more energy than light ones. There are also substantial variations between apparently similar individuals. Measuring the energy cost of different activities for people with different body weights is very time consuming. Instead the energy used for a particular physical activity can be calculated by multiplying the BMR by a factor appropriate to that activity. This factor, the *physical activity ratio* (PAR), is calculated as follows:

$$PAR = \frac{\text{the energy cost of an activity per minute}}{\text{the energy cost of the BMR per minute}}$$

Thus the energy cost for sitting at rest is 1.2 x BMR; for walking at a normal pace 4 x BMR; for jogging 7 x BMR, etc. By combining all these activities over a 24-hour period, a multiple of the BMR, which characterises a person's lifestyle, can be derived. This multiple - the *physical activity level* (PAL) - is calculated as follows:

$$PAL = \frac{\text{the total energy required over 24 hours}}{\text{the BMR over 24 hours}}$$

Daily energy expenditure can be estimated by multiplying BMR by PAL. A PAL of 1.4, representing very little physical activity at work or during leisure time, applies to most people in the UK. Values for PAL of 1.6 for women and 1.7 for men represent moderate activity during work time and leisure; PAL values of 1.8 for women and 1.9 for men represent high levels of activity at work and during recreation.

Some examples of the energy expended on activities by an average 25-year-old woman office worker weighing 62 kg (10 stone) are shown below:

	Average energy expenditure	
	(kJ/min)	(kcal/min)
Everyday activities		
Sitting, eating	5	1.1
Standing, cooking	9	2.1
Washing and dressing	9	2.1
Walking moderately quickly	15	3.5
Walking up and down stairs	28	6.5
Work and recreation		
Office, sitting	6	1.5
Office, walking slowly	11	2.6
Dancing	19	4.5
Average jogging	27	6.5

Total energy requirements

The dietary energy required by an individual who is neither gaining nor losing weight exactly equals the energy expended on maintenance and physical activity. In practice this balance is achieved over periods of a few days, with remarkable accuracy: an intake of only 40 kJ (10 kcal) in excess of expenditure each day would be equivalent to a weight gain of about 0.5 kg (1 lb) every year. The energy expended during a day can be estimated from the BMR and the average PAR values for various activities, taking into account the time spent on each. A male sedentary worker, such as a civil servant, with a moderately active leisure time, might expend 10.9 MJ (2633 kcal) in a typical day as shown in the table on next page.

The example used is of a man 40 years old, weighing 76 kg and having a BMR of 7.3 MJ per day. His physical activity level (PAL) would be 1.5 (Total energy expenditure divided by BMR). Because of individual variations, the diet of any particular sedentary worker may provide more or less energy than this; the average intake of a group of such people would, however, be expected to be close to this value. In summary, the daily energy requirement of any adult is that amount which maintains the desirable body weight.

BODY SIZE AND COMPOSITION

Heavy people use more energy for maintenance and physical activity, although some may spend less time than lighter people in activities. Women tend to need less energy than men, although their needs are increased during the last months of pregnancy and during lactation.

	PAR	Average energy expenditure	
		(MJ)	(kcal)
8 h asleep	1.0	2.4	576
8 h at work			
6½ h sitting	1.4	2.7	652
1½ h standing and slow walking	1.8	0.8	194
8 h non-occupational activities			
15 min washing and dressing	2.5	0.2	45
2 h 15 min commuting	1.7	1.1	273
1½ h light domestic chores	2.2	1.0	273
3 h sitting, eating, reading, watching TV	1.2	1.1	258
30 min squash	7.5	1.1	273
30 min light gardening	3.5	0.5	125
Total energy expenditure (TEE)		10.9	2633

AGE

Requirements for maintenance are proportionately highest in infants and young children, and usually lowest in elderly people who have less lean body tissue and are less active.

PHYSICAL ACTIVITY

The degree of activity is the most important factor in determining energy requirements, and also the most difficult to assess. Sedentary workers (for example, those who spend most of their time at an office desk or behind the wheel of a motor vehicle) need a total of about 3.8 MJ (900 kcal) for 8 hours work; moderately active people (many industrial workers, nursing staff and postal workers) need about 5.0 MJ (1200 kcal), and very active workers (oil rig workers, building labourers, farm workers, fishing crews and armed forces recruits) have an average need for about 7.5 MJ (1800 kcal) during 8 hours at work. Leisure activities such as jogging, particularly if indulged in regularly or for long periods, also affect the day's requirements.

GROWTH, PREGNANCY AND LACTATION

Additional energy is needed during growth to provide for the extra body tissue. In newborn infants, about one-third of the total energy needs is used for laying down new tissue. However, this falls to about 4 per cent of total energy needs by one year of age and even in the rapidly growing child this need remains small in comparison with the requirement for maintenance and movement.

During pregnancy and lactation (breastfeeding), all the infant's needs for energy (as for other nutrients, see p. 124) must be supplied by the mother. Extra food energy is needed during the final months of pregnancy (0.8 MJ (200 kcal) per day during the last trimester). Some of this is used to build up a store of about 2 kg of fat in the mother, which may be gradually drawn upon during lactation, but an additional intake of 1.9 - 2.4 MJ (450 - 570 kcal) per day from the diet is also recommended from the start of lactation to three months onwards (p. 77).

Obesity

The 2003 Health Survey for England classified well over half of all adults as either overweight or obese. In England, 22.2% of men and 23.0% of women were obese i.e. with a Body Mass Index (see below) over 30. In 1993 the figures were 13.2% and 16.4%, respectively. The prevalence of obesity has trebled since 1980 and, according to the National Audit Office, there is no sign that this trend is moderating. In Wales and Scotland 18% and 24%, respectively of adults were classified as obese in 2003/04. The increase in childhood obesity has also been marked; the prevalence increased among the under 11 age group in England from 9.9% in 1995 to 13.7% in 2003. Obese people have a greater risk of developing diseases that include diabetes (see p. 132), cardiovascular disease, high blood pressure and some cancers.

If individuals eat or drink foods which provide more energy than they use up in their daily activities, some of the fat, protein, carbohydrate or alcohol will be converted into body fat, the most readily convertible nutrient being fat. Any kind of food can therefore be 'fattening' if eaten in a quantity that results in energy intake in excess of expenditure. Some foods, however, are more concentrated sources of energy than others. These tend to be foods containing little water and a high proportion of fat, such as butter, margarine, fatty meat, fried foods, ice cream, cakes and biscuits. High palatability of foods can also encourage excessive amounts to be eaten. Obesity may occur even if energy intake is only slightly greater than output if it is consistently so over a long period of time.

The broad range of weights found for people at different heights has been used to construct the chart shown in Figure 1. This can be used to indicate whether an individual is an acceptable weight for their height. The Body Mass Index (BMI), calculated as weight in kilograms divided by the square of the height in metres, is also used to assess the degree to which a person is overweight. A BMI of 18.5 or below is underweight; 18.5 - 24.9 is desirable; 25 - 29.9 is overweight; and 30 or above is considered obese[1]. Whereas BMI is a measure of general obesity, waist circumference and waist-to-hip ratios provide measures of central obesity, which has a stronger relationship with the risk of chronic diseases than does general obesity or

---

[1] A quick BMI calculator can be found at www.eatwell.gov.uk/healthydiet/healthyweight/bmicalculator

BMI. A raised waist circumference of 94 cm or more for men or 80 cm or more for women or a waist-to-hip ratio of more than 1.0 (generally known as 'apple' shape) indicates increased risk of diseases such as heart disease. Those people who carry more weight around their hips, with less risk of heart disease, are generally known as 'pear' shaped[2].

Weight may be lost by decreasing energy intake or increasing physical activity or both. Conversely, weight may be gained by increasing energy intake, or decreasing physical activity or both. The exact consequences of these changes are difficult to predict because of the large differences between individual responses and some measure of adaptation, but for many people the part played by changes in activity may be comparatively small. For example, if a man trying to lose weight takes a brisk half-hour walk, he will expend about 420 kJ (100 kcal) more than if he sat watching television. If at the end of his walk, however, he is thirsty and drinks a pint of beer, he will take in substantially more energy than he used up. If this happens frequently he should not be surprised if his weight increases. Nevertheless, *regular* vigorous exercise can be an important factor in weight control.

---

[2] An easy way for someone to check if they are apple shaped and have too much weight around their middle is the Ashwell chart found at : www.eatwell.gov.uk/healthydiet/healthyweight/yourbodyshape/

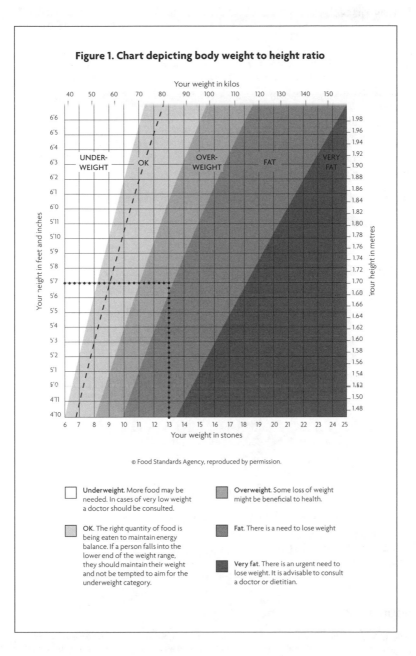

Figure 1. Chart depicting body weight to height ratio

Your weight in kilos

Your height in feet and inches

Your height in metres

Your weight in stones

© Food Standards Agency, reproduced by permission.

Underweight. More food may be needed. In cases of very low weight a doctor should be consulted.

OK. The right quantity of food is being eaten to maintain energy balance. If a person falls into the lower end of the weight range, they should maintain their weight and not be tempted to aim for the underweight category.

Overweight. Some loss of weight might be beneficial to health.

Fat. There is a need to lose weight

Very fat. There is an urgent need to lose weight. It is advisable to consult a doctor or dietitian.

Eating disorders

It is important to realise that some body fat is essential for health, but some people, particularly teenage girls, seek to reduce their weight below the desirable range shown in Figure 1. *Anorexia nervosa* and *bulimia nervosa* are psychological conditions expressed by extremes of behaviour involving food avoidance or alternate binge-eating and vomiting, respectively, and can be fatal.

Energy value of food

The energy provided by the fat, protein and carbohydrate in food, and by alcohol, can be measured. Taking into account the small proportions of these macronutrients which are not absorbed into the body:

1 g dietary carbohydrate (calculated as monosaccharides) provides 16 kJ or 3.75 kcal
1 g dietary fat provides 37 kJ or 9 kcal
1 g dietary protein provides 17 kJ or 4 kcal
1 g alcohol provides 29 kJ or 7 kcal.

Polyols also provide energy (see p. 6) and small amounts of energy can be derived from organic acids such as citric acid in fruits and drinks and acetic acid in vinegar, with each gram providing approximately 13 kJ (3 kcal). The micronutrients (minerals and vitamins); fibre and water do not provide energy.

The energy value of any food can be calculated when the proportions of the nutrients in it are known. For example, if 100 g of potato crisps contain 49.3 g carbohydrate, 37.6 g fat and 5.6 g protein, the energy content is calculated as follows:

	49.3 x 16	= 788.8 kJ from carbohydrate
	37.6 x 37	= 1391.2 kJ from fat
	5.6 x 17	= 95.2 kJ from protein
	Total	2275.2 kJ
or	49.3 x 3.75	= 184.9 kcal from carbohydrate
	37.6 x 9	= 338.4 kcal from fat
	5.6 x 4	= 22.4 kcal from protein
	Total	545.7 kcal

It is misleading, however, to imply that energy values can be obtained with such precision; decimal points should not be included in the results, which might be rounded to 2275 kJ or 546 kcal. But when performing further calculations such as for the proportion of energy derived from fat, it is wiser to use the detailed figures and round off only at the end (see also Appendix 4):

$$\frac{1391.2}{2275.2} \times 100 = 61.15 \text{ or 61 per cent of energy from fat}$$

Sources of energy in the diet

Nearly all the weight of any food is made up of protein, fat and carbohydrate together with water. Foods which contain large amounts of water, such as salad vegetables, fruit and clear soups will contain little protein, fat or carbohydrate, and consequently provide little energy. In contrast, dry foods such as breakfast cereals, and foods rich in fat and sugar are concentrated sources of energy. The main sources of energy in the UK diet are cereals and cereal products, which include foods like bread, breakfast cereals, biscuits and cakes, which provide a third of energy intake on average. Bread alone provides 13%. Meat and meat products provide 15% of energy intake, milk and milk products 10%, drinks including alcoholic drinks 10% and potatoes and savoury snacks 9%.

The energy (and water) contents of selected foods are shown in Table 7.

Table 7. Average energy value and water content of selected foods (edible portion)

	Energy		Water
	(kJ/100 g)	(kcal/100 g)	(g/100g)
Milk, whole	274	66	88
Milk, semi-skimmed	195	46	90
Milk, skimmed	136	32	91
Cheese, Cheddar	1725	416	37
Yogurt, low-fat, fruit	331	78	79
Beef, stewing steak (lean and fat), stewed	852	203	59
Bacon, streaky, fried	1389	335	45
Chicken, roast, meat, average	742	177	65
Cod, fillet, baked	408	96	77
Fish fingers, grilled	838	200	56
Sardines, canned in oil	918	220	59
Eggs, chicken, boiled	612	147	75
Butter	3059	744	15
Fat spread (40% fat), not polyunsaturated	1519	368	52
Vegetable oil, blended	3696	899	0
Sugar, white	1680	394	0
Courgettes, boiled	81	19	93
Lettuce	59	14	95
Carrots, old, boiled	100	24	91
Potatoes, old, boiled	306	72	80
Chips, fried in vegetable oil, takeaway	1001	239	52
Apples, eating, raw	199	47	85
Banana	403	95	75
Orange	158	37	86
Raisins	1159	272	13
Bread, white	931	219	39
Bread, wholemeal	922	217	41
Biscuits, chocolate, full coated	2105	501	1
Cornflakes	1601	376	3
Crispbread, rye	1312	308	6
Lager	121	29	93
Wine, white, medium	308	74	86
Spirits	919	222	68

6 Digestion of food and absorption of major nutrients

Food has been defined as any solid or liquid which, when swallowed, can provide the body with energy, or material for growth and repair, or certain substances for regulating body processes. However, it is clear that almost any food can be recovered virtually intact from the stomach if vomiting occurs soon after it is eaten. Therefore, food cannot really be said to have entered the body until it has been:

(a) *digested*, i.e. physically and chemically broken down into simple component parts which can be
(b) *absorbed*, i.e. passed through the walls of the digestive tract into the blood (or lymph)

Flavour and appetite

For food to be eaten, it must be appetizing or we must be hungry - preferably both circumstances should apply. When and how much we eat is determined by a number of complex factors. The sensation of *hunger* occurs when levels of glucose and fatty acids in the blood are reduced and the stomach is empty. But people, especially obese people, do not eat only when they are hungry or stop when they cease to feel hungry. *Appetite* is a sensation which relates to the smell and taste of particular foods and their ingredients, and is influenced by the surroundings, habits and emotional state of the individual, all of which can also increase or decrease the flow of saliva and other digestive juices. Thus, where there is freedom of choice, more attractive foods are likely to be eaten in preference to others, and it can be seen that good cooking and pleasant surroundings are important in nutrition. It should, however, be noted that some appetizing foods such as confectionery products can be relatively low in many nutrients, and that unappetizing foods can provide nourishment - as when an unconscious person is fed through a naso-gastric tube.

The process of digestion

Although cooking softens meat fibres and the cellulose of plant materials, and gelatinises starch, true digestion only begins when food enters the mouth and digestive tract. The digestive tract, illustrated in Figure 2, is basically a tube about 5 m long.

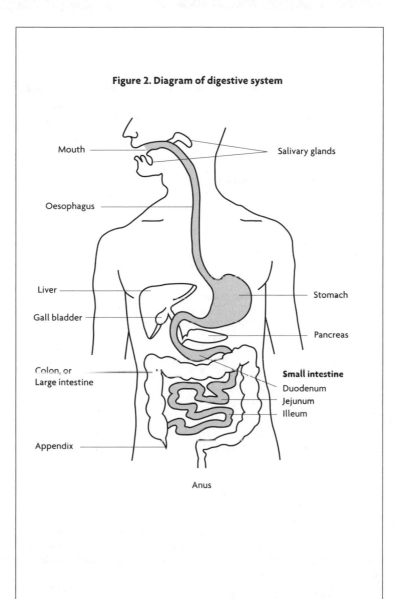

Figure 2. Diagram of digestive system

Mouth

Salivary glands

Oesophagus

Liver

Stomach

Gall bladder

Pancreas

Colon, or
Large intestine

Small intestine

Duodenum

Jejunum

Illeum

Appendix

Anus

IN THE MOUTH

(a) Food is mechanically broken down by chewing. It is therefore important to have healthy teeth and gums.
(b) The food is mixed and moistened with saliva.

Saliva comes from salivary glands under the tongue and at the back of the mouth. It is usually present in the mouth, but its flow is increased by the smell and taste of food and by chewing. It helps the food to be swallowed, and also contains an enzyme, salivary *amylase*, which converts a small amount of the starch into maltose.

IN THE STOMACH

After the mixture of food particles and saliva has been swallowed - the final voluntary action - it takes about 3 seconds to pass down the oesophagus into the stomach, where:

(a) the food is mixed with gastric juice
(b) more mechanical breakdown results from stomach contractions.

Gastric juice is produced by the lining of the stomach in response to the same stimuli that increase saliva flow. Normally, about 3 litres are produced each day. It has three important constituents:

(a) the enzyme *pepsin*, which begins the digestion of protein,
(b) about 0.2 to 0.4 per cent of hydrochloric acid (much more acid than in 'acid foods') that destroys most of the bacteria which could be present in food and water and provides the acid conditions necessary for the pepsin to be active,
(c) 'intrinsic factor', necessary for subsequent absorption of vitamin B_{12}.

Speed of digestion in the stomach
The main function of the stomach is to act as a reservoir: digestion still proceeds if the stomach is completely removed. Food normally remains in the stomach for 2 to 4 hours before the resulting semi-liquid mixture (chyme) is passed little by little into the small intestine. The exact time taken for food to pass depends on the emotional state of the person and the type of food eaten: foods rich in carbohydrate (such as rice) pass most quickly and those rich in fat most slowly.

IN THE SMALL INTESTINE

Despite its name, the small intestine is the longest part of the digestive tract. It is about 3 m in length (although because of the loss of tone and elasticity, it is found to be 7 - 8 m long after death), compared with about 1 m for the large intestine. It is, however, only 2 - 4 cm in diameter compared with 6 cm for the latter. The first distinct part of the small intestine is called the *duodenum*; the remainder consists of the *jejunum* and finally the *ileum*. It is in the small intestine that the main part of both digestion and absorption takes place.

In the duodenum, the digestive juices poured on to the food mixture from three sources are:

(a) *bile*, which is produced in the liver and stored in the gall bladder. Bile salts emulsify the fat into microscopic droplets so that it can be digested.
(b) *pancreatic juice*, from the pancreas. This alkaline liquid neutralizes the acid chyme, and contains a number of enzymes for breaking down fats, proteins and carbohydrates into their component parts. The most important of these are *lipase* which splits fatty acids from triglycerides of fat, *trypsin* and *chymotrypsin* which split proteins into small peptides and amino acids, and amylase which splits starch into maltose.
(c) *intestinal juice*, from the walls of the small intestine itself. This also contains digestive enzymes.

The final phase of digestion occurs *in* the intestinal wall after absorption, when peptides are split into their component amino acids, maltose is converted into glucose by *maltase*, sucrose into glucose and fructose by *sucrase*, and lactose into glucose and galactose by *lactase*. A summary of the major enzymes of digestion is provided in Table 8.

Table 8. Summary of the major enzymes of digestion

Enzyme	Where active	Action
Salivary amylase	Mouth	Some starch to maltose
Pepsin	Stomach	Protein to peptides
Rennin (in infants only)	Stomach	Milk protein to peptides
Trypsin (from pancreas)	Intestine	Protein to peptides and amino acids
Chymotrypsin (from pancreas)	Intestine	Protein to peptides and amino acids
Lipase (from pancreas and intestine)	Intestine	Fat to fatty acids
Amylase (from pancreas)	Intestine	Starch (and glycogen) to maltose
Maltase	Intestinal wall	Maltose to glucose
Sucrase	Intestinal wall	Sucrose to glucose and fructose
Lactase	Intestinal wall	Lactose to glucose and galactose

IN THE LARGE INTESTINE
Substances which have resisted digestion and absorption thus far can be used for food by the bacteria present in the large intestine (colon). Some cellulose and other components of fibre may then be broken down, and the bacteria will form B-vitamins and vitamin K which provide small amounts of additional nutrients for absorption. They also generate gas (mainly hydrogen).

DIGESTION IN INFANTS
Before birth, infants are nourished through their bloodstream via the mother's placenta. The change to intestinal digestion does not develop fully for several months after birth. Three consequences in particular may be noted:

(a) for a few days, some whole proteins can be absorbed without digestion. In this way, antibodies against some diseases may be absorbed intact from the mother's milk.
(b) the stomach contains the enzyme *rennin*, which clots the casein of milk and begins its digestion.
(c) starch cannot readily be digested until the infant is several months old.

INDIGESTION

A food or food component is indigestible if it cannot be fully broken down into substances capable of absorption. Some, such as lactose from milk in lactose-intolerant individuals, will reach the large intestine and be fermented by the bacteria present; this results in the production of gas and diarrhoea. Indigestion also means discomfort or pain in the gastro-intestinal tract resulting from eating. It can result as much from emotional factors as from the passage of indigestible foods.

The process of absorption

IN THE MOUTH

No significant absorption occurs through the lining of the mouth.

IN THE STOMACH

The following simple substances can pass through the lining of the stomach into the blood stream in small quantities:

(a) water
(b) alcohol
(c) sugars
(d) minerals which are soluble in water, such as sodium chloride (salt)
(e) vitamins which are soluble in water, i.e. B-vitamins (but not vitamin B_{12}, which can only be absorbed in the ileum with the aid of the intrinsic factor produced by the stomach) and vitamin C.

IN THE SMALL INTESTINE

Almost all the absorption of nutrients occurs through the walls of the small intestine. Most of the water, alcohol, simple sugars, minerals and water-soluble vitamins are absorbed here too, as well as the digestion products of the energy-producing nutrients. These are:

(a) peptides and amino acids from proteins,
(b) fatty acids from fats,
(c) disaccharides from starch.

Fat-soluble vitamins are absorbed in association with the fatty acids.

Absorption into the cells of the intestinal wall is remarkably efficient; indeed, more than half of the small intestine can be removed without major consequences. The surface of the wall contains innumerable projections, called *villi*, which present a very large surface area (20 - 40 m² in total) for absorption. This process occurs both passively (by diffusion) and actively (when specific nutrients are drawn into cells already containing large amounts of those nutrients).

Absorption can, however, be impaired. In coeliac disease the villi are lost. Substances such as laxatives and fibre which speed the passage of the intestinal contents may reduce absorption in general. The fibre and phytic acid present in wholemeal cereals may also reduce the absorption of specific minerals including calcium, iron and zinc.

IN THE LARGE INTESTINE

The main functions of the large intestine are to absorb water from the residue moving through it from the small intestine, and to store the resultant faeces until they are expelled through the anus. Faeces are 70 - 80 per cent water, but also contain the undigested materials of food. The solid portion consists of fibre, debris from the continuously replaced cells of the intestinal wall including intestinal bacteria, and a small amount of undigested food. The entire passage of food from mouth to anus takes from 1 to 3 days, but it can be decreased by disease or by antibiotics which kill the intestinal bacteria, or it can be increased to as long as a week by diets very low in fibre.

The fate of major nutrients in the body

CARBOHYDRATES

The disaccharides entering the intestinal wall are split into monosaccharides which are carried by the bloodstream directly to the liver. They may then be:

(a) delivered as glucose to all the cells of the body to be used directly for energy via a series of controlled steps which produce carbon dioxide and water

(b) converted into glycogen and stored in the liver and skeletal muscles as a readily available source of energy

(c) converted into fatty acids and stored in the body fat (adipose tissue) as a source of energy.

The hormone *insulin* is required for the cellular metabolism of glucose (see diabetes, page 132), but fructose and dietary sorbitol (which is converted in the body into fructose) do not require insulin for their metabolism.

FATS

Almost all the fatty acids which enter the intestinal wall are immediately rebuilt into triglycerides which are carried to the bloodstream by lymph. Fat, in the form of microscopic particles called *chylomicrons*, circulates in the blood plasma which has a milky appearance for some time after a large meal is eaten. When fat reaches tissues requiring energy, fatty acids are released from it by enzymes and taken up into the cells. Fat may be further transformed by the liver, and most is finally deposited in the adipose tissue. Dietary fat is more easily converted into body fat than is the carbohydrate in food. The body's reservoir of fat is constantly available as a source of energy via another series of controlled steps which also give rise to carbon dioxide and water.

PROTEINS

When the peptides enter the intestinal wall they are split into amino acids which are carried in the blood directly to the liver. They may then be:

(a) passed into the general circulation where they enter the body's 'pool' of indispensable and dispensable amino acids. These are then built into the structural proteins and specific enzymes which each cell needs.
(b) converted into those amino acids which are in short supply
(c) oxidized for energy, in some cases after conversion into glucose, if there is a residual excess of amino acids. Urea is also formed and excreted through the kidneys. If the diet as a whole is inadequate in energy, then a greater proportion of the protein will be used for this purpose in order to keep the body alive.

Control of nutrients in the blood

Blood is the means by which most nutrients are carried to and from the cells where they are needed. The concentration of most nutrients in the blood is normally controlled automatically as described in Chapters 7 and 8. In addition, when carbohydrate is eaten, the resulting slight increase in blood glucose is soon reduced by the hormone insulin. In *diabetes*, however, the blood glucose levels are not kept within the normal range. In the case of Type I or insulin-dependent diabetes, the pancreas does not secrete sufficient insulin, and the blood glucose concentration increases until the excess is excreted by the kidneys into the urine. This imbalance is so severe that insulin must be injected. Type II or non insulin-dependent diabetes occurs when the tissues develop resistance to the effects of insulin. It is strongly related to overweight and low physical activity as well as genetic predisposition. This form of diabetes can often be controlled by dietary regulation. The prevalence of Type II diabetes is increasing among adults in the UK as the incidence of overweight and obesity increases, and is now found in children in whom it was previously rarely seen. Dietary advice for people with diabetes is similar to that for the population in general: maintenance of a healthy weight and consumption of a diet that is:

- low in fat (particularly saturated fat)
- low in sugars
- low in salt
- high in fruit and vegetables (at least 5 portions a day). However, drinking large amounts of fruit juice could cause problems with controlling blood sugar for some people with diabetes, because of the high fruit sugar (fructose) it contains;
- high in starchy carbohydrate foods (especially wholegrain types) such as bread, chapatti, rice, pasta, potatoes and yams. These should form the base of meals.

There are no foods that people with diabetes should never eat. Nor do they need to cut out all sugars. However, people with diabetes should try to eat only small amounts of foods that are high in fat and sugar, or both. Cakes and biscuits can be eaten sparingly, as part of a balanced diet.

The Food Standards Agency and Diabetes UK (formerly the British Diabetic Association) don't recommend products aimed at diabetics. Foods that are labelled 'diabetic' are not necessarily healthier or more suitable for diabetics than other foods. They also tend to be more expensive than other products.

7 Minerals

Most if not all of the inorganic elements or minerals can be detected in the body, but only about 15 of them are known to be essential and must be derived from food. Minute amounts of a further five or more are necessary for normal life in other animal species, and may well prove to be necessary for humans; it is difficult, however, to conceive of a dietary deficiency of these. Minerals have three main functions:

(a) as constituents of the bones and teeth. These include *calcium, phosphorus* and *magnesium*.
(b) as soluble salts which help to control the composition of body fluids and cells. These include *sodium* and *chloride* in the fluids outside the cells (e.g. blood), and *potassium*, magnesium and phosphorus inside the cells.
(c) as essential adjuncts to many enzymes, and other proteins such as haemoglobin, which are necessary for the release and utilisation of energy. *Iron*, phosphorus and *zinc*, and most of the other elements described at the end of this chapter, act in this way.

The elements mentioned above are in general needed in the greatest amounts in the diet or are present in the largest amounts in the body tissues (Table 9); with the exception of zinc, these, together with sulphur which is mainly present as part of the amino acids methionine and cysteine, are generally considered as the *major minerals*. The remainder, including zinc, chromium, cobalt, copper, fluoride, iodine, manganese, molybdenum and selenium, are equally important but are needed, or are present in the body tissues, in smaller quantities. They are called *trace elements*. The amounts of selected elements needed to maintain the health of various age groups in the population are discussed in Chapter 9. However, many minerals and trace elements can be toxic in excess. In 2003 the Expert Group on Vitamins and Minerals (EVM), an independent advisory committee, was asked by the UK Government to advise on the safety of intakes of minerals used in food supplements and fortified foods (see reference in Appendix 9). The Group's recommendations for levels of minerals and trace elements taken as supplements each day that are unlikely to be harmful are given in each of the following sections.

Table 9. Daily intake and total body content of minerals for an adult man

	Daily intake[a]	Total body content[d]
Major minerals		
Calcium	0.9 g	1200 g[e]
Iron	13 mg	4.2 g
Magnesium	0.3 g	19 g
Phosphorus	1.3 g	780 g
Potassium	3.0 g	140 g
Sodium	3.8 g	140 g
Trace elements		
Chromium	0.1[b] mg	Less than 2 mg
Cobalt	0.01[c] mg	1.5 mg
Copper	1.48 mg	72 mg
Fluoride	1.2[b] mg	2.6 g
Iodine	220 µg	13 mg
Manganese	3.4 mg	12 mg
Selenium	40[c] µg	>15 mg
Zinc	9.2 mg	2.3 g

[a] From all sources. Unless otherwise indicated values for the years 2000-01 from National Diet and Nutrition Survey: adults aged 19 to 64 years. Vol. 3, 2003.
[b] Total Diet Study, 1997. Intakes of fluoride may be much higher in those people who drink large volumes of tea made with fluoridated water.
[c] Total Diet study, 1994.
[d] Manual of Nutrition, 10th edition.
[e] Expert Group on Vitamins and Minerals. Food Standards Agency, 2003.
Intakes are likely to be far greater than requirements. A variable proportion is actually absorbed into the body (ranging from almost 100 per cent for sodium and chloride down to 5-10 per cent for iron, copper, manganese and probably chromium and cobalt too); the amount absorbed normally balances the amount lost in urine and sweat, except where increased retention is necessary during growth.

Major minerals

IRON

Function, and effects of deficiency
The healthy adult body contains 3 - 4 g of iron, more than half of which is in the form of haemoglobin, the red pigment of blood. Iron is also present in the muscle protein myoglobin, and is stored to some extent in organs such as the liver. This store is an important source of iron for the first six months of an infant's life because the amount of iron in milk is small. Iron plays a major part in the body's use of oxygen: haemoglobin transports oxygen from the lungs to the tissues, and other iron-containing substances utilise the oxygen within the cells.

In Britain the average adult daily iron intake from food in 2000-01 was about 13 mg for men and 10 mg for women. These values are above the Reference Nutrient Intake (p. 78) for men, but below that for women, many of whom have increased iron needs due to menstrual blood losses. Adult women were reported to obtain, on average, 16 per cent of their total intake from dietary supplements, but men obtained most of their iron from food and only 6% from supplements. On average about 25% of women, but only 1% of men had intakes from food below the Lower Reference Nutrient Intake (p. 77). If food provides insufficient iron to replace the body's losses, the stores are gradually depleted. Eventually, anaemia results. Anaemia can also arise from a number of other causes including deficiencies of folic acid and vitamin B_{12} (p. 66 and 67); treatment is best effected medically and not nutritionally, for example by the use of iron supplements.

Absorption and excretion
The amount of iron in the body is controlled almost entirely by the amount absorbed, because losses occur only when blood or other whole cells are lost in the general wear and tear of life. Losses do not occur at the end of the red blood cell's life of 3 - 4 months, because the iron from them is efficiently re-utilised.

The iron in the diet exists in two forms – *haem* and *non-haem* iron. About ninety per cent of the iron in the British diet is made up of non-haem iron (iron salts) and about ten per cent is haem iron from the red pigments of meat and offals. The extent to which iron is absorbed depends on the form in which it occurs. The amount of non-haem iron absorbed is very variable and is influenced by the body's iron status and by the combination of foods ingested. Absorption of haem iron is relatively good (20 - 30 per cent) and not influenced by these factors. The non-haem iron occurring in cereals, pulses, vegetables, fruits, and dairy products is generally less well absorbed, but absorption increases when the body's stores are depleted and when needs are greatest, as in growing children or menstruating or pregnant women. Its absorption also depends on other factors in the diet. It is increased by the presence of meat, poultry or fish, and may also be increased by sources of vitamin C, such as citrus fruits, fruit juices, green leafy vegetables and salad items like tomatoes and sweet peppers, when these are eaten at the same time as the source of non-haem iron. Absorption may be decreased by the tannins in tea and by some forms of fibre. The iron in eggs is largely unavailable. If women have heavy periods, extra iron may need to be prescribed by a GP.

Sources and intakes
In Britain, all wheat flour, other than wholemeal, is fortified with iron by law (p. 104). Other foods are fortified voluntarily by manufacturers. About forty per cent of the iron in the British diet comes from cereals and cereal products, with twenty percent from breakfast cereals alone, about seventeen per cent comes from meat and meat products and about ten percent from vegetables, not including potatoes. The total amounts of iron present in selected foods are shown in Table 10.

Most people should be able to get all the iron they need by eating a varied and balanced diet. Iron supplements should not be taken in high doses as too much can cause gastrointestinal problems. Guidance suggests that taking 17 mg or less of iron as supplements a day is unlikely to be harmful. If a higher dose is being taken under medical advice then this should be continued.

Table 10. Total iron content of selected foods (edible portion)

	(mg/100 g)		(mg/100 g)
Milk, semi-skimmed	0.02	Potatoes, old, boiled	0.4
Eggs, chicken, boiled	1.9	Watercress	2.2
Beef, stewing steak, stewed	2.3	Okra, boiled	0.6
Beefburgers, grilled	2.5	Apricots, semi-dried, as eaten	3.4
Chicken, roast, meat only, average	0.8	Bananas	0.3
Kidney, pig's, stewed	6.4	Bread, white	1.6
Liver, lamb's, fried	7.7	Bread, wholemeal	2.4
Liver pate	5.9	Cornflakes, fortified	7.9
Cod, fillet, baked	0.1	Curry powder	58.3
Sardines, in tomato sauce	2.9	Soy sauce	2.4
Broccoli, boiled	1.0	Cocoa powder	10.5
Lettuce	0.7	Chocolate, plain	2.3
Cabbage, boiled	0.3	Chocolate, milk	1.4
Lentils, green, dried, boiled	3.5	Wine, red	0.9
Red kidney beans, dried, boiled	2.5	Wine, white, dry	0.5
		Spirits	0.0

The main sources of iron in the diet are cereals and cereal products (especially breakfast cereals and white bread), meat and meat products, and vegetables (excluding potatoes).

CALCIUM

Function

Calcium is the most abundant mineral in the body. All but about 1 per cent of it occurs in the bones and teeth, together with more than three-quarters of the body's phosphorus, in the form of calcium phosphates deposited in an organic framework. In addition to giving strength to the bones, these minerals act as a reserve supply for other needs and the calcium is constantly withdrawn into and replaced from the blood at carefully controlled rates. The remaining 5 -10 g of calcium are essential for the contraction of muscles, including the heart muscle, for nerve function, for the activity of several enzymes, and for normal clotting of the blood.

The effects of deficiency

Rickets and osteomalacia

Too little calcium in the bodies of young children results in stunted growth and in rickets (where the leg bones are deformed). In adults, the deficiency may show as osteomalacia (decalcified bones). The primary deficiency in rickets and osteomalacia, however, is of vitamin D so that too little calcium is absorbed. It occurs among some ethnic groups and in elderly people (especially those who are housebound) who remain indoors or wear enveloping clothes. Such people have a low exposure to sunlight and consequently form little or no vitamin D in their skin (p. 72). They may also be eating diets low in calcium or high in phytate (see below). Women who lose large quantities of calcium through repeated pregnancies and lactation are also at risk of osteomalacia.

Osteoporosis

Osteoporosis is a reduction of bone density and strength that causes bones to become brittle and fracture easily, and is caused by progressive loss of bone components as people age. Bone density increases until it reaches a Peak Bone Mass at around the age of 30. The extent of Peak Bone Mass depends on how well nourished young people have been during childhood and early adulthood. As people age beyond 30 their bone density decreases. This decline is particularly rapid in women about the time of the menopause. The most common sites of osteoporotic fracture are the vertebrae (resulting in curvature of the spine), wrist and hip. This condition causes a great deal of suffering, particularly for elderly women, and can result in the loss of independence. The resulting health care required for the elderly is also costly for the health services.

The causes of osteoporosis are multi-factorial. Lifestyle factors, such as diet and exercise, play an important role and are amenable to change so may help people reduce their risk of fracture. Studies are continuing into the role of nutrition, but the importance of calcium and vitamin D (see p. 72) for bone health has been known for some time. There is increasing evidence that fruit and vegetables may be important in reducing the risk of fracture later in life. A healthy balanced diet along with weight-bearing physical activity, such as brisk walking, spending time outdoors to encourage vitamin D formation in the skin (see p. 72) and the avoidance of smoking seem to promote healthy bones.

Other possible protective effects of calcium

It is thought that calcium may help to lower high blood pressure and may help to protect against colon and breast cancer, although more evidence is needed to support this.

Absorption and excretion

Only 30 - 40 per cent of the calcium in the diet is normally absorbed and the remainder is lost in the faeces. But without adequate amounts of vitamin D, little or no calcium can be absorbed, and when fibre or phytic acid (present mainly in the outer layers of cereals) or oxalate (present in spinach and rhubarb) is added to the diet, calcium absorption is also reduced. It was partly to compensate for this that calcium carbonate was added to the high-extraction flour used during and after World War II; it is still added to all flour except wholemeal although it is now known that the body can adapt to the presence of phytic acid.

Excretion of absorbed calcium is mainly through the kidneys, and is increased when the diet contains large amounts of protein; some calcium is also lost in sweat. Adults normally absorb enough calcium to balance these losses until middle age unless they are immobilized, but lactating women, and growing children who are forming new bone, must consume more.

Sources and intakes

Few foods besides milk, yogurt and cheese and, in the UK, most breads contain significant amounts of calcium. It is therefore important that these foods are included in the diet, especially for children and adolescents. Reduced-fat milks contain essentially the same quantity of calcium as whole milk (see Table 11). However, children below the age of two need an energy-dense diet and should always be given whole milk as a main drink.

Most people should be able to get all the calcium they need by eating a varied and balanced diet. No additional intake is considered necessary for pregnancy, although an increase is recommended during lactation. The average adult intake of calcium from food in Britain is nearly 900 mg per day, which is adequate for the needs of most people. Adult men and women consumed on average about 1000 and 780 mg per day, respectively, from food in 2000-01. Dietary supplements contribute about an additional ten per cent of calcium intake in women over fifty, but little on average to other adult population groups. If calcium supplements are taken, it is important that excessive amounts are not taken as this could be harmful. Guidance suggests that taking 1500 mg or less of calcium a day in the form of supplements is unlikely to cause any adverse effects.

Table 11. Calcium content of selected foods (edible portion)

	(mg/100 g)		(mg/100 g)
Milk, whole	118	Courgettes, boiled	19
Milk, semi-skimmed	120	Cabbage, boiled	33
Milk, skimmed	122	Okra, boiled	120
Milk, dried, skimmed	1280	Onions, fried	47
Yogurt, low fat, fruit	140	Potatoes, old, boiled	5
Fromage frais, plain	110	Watercress, raw	170
Cheese, Cheddar	739	Apples (eating)	4
Cheese, cottage	127	Oranges	47
Ice cream, non-dairy	72	Raisins	46
Eggs, boiled (chicken)	57	Peanuts, dry, roasted	52
Beef, stewing steak, stewed	15	Bread, white	177
Cod, fillet, baked	11	Bread, wholemeal	106
Sardines - canned in oil, drained	500	Rice, white, boiled	18
Baked beans	53		

The main sources of calcium in the diet are milk and milk products (especially semi-skimmed milk and cheese), and cereals and cereal products (especially white bread). For some people, hard water and the bones in canned sardines and salmon can be important.

PHOSPHORUS

Phosphorus is the second most abundant mineral in the body and, in the form of various phosphates, has a wide variety of essential functions. Calcium phosphates provide the strength of the bones and teeth, and inorganic phosphates are a major constituent of all cells. Phosphates play an essential role in the liberation and utilisation of energy from food. They are also constituents of nucleic acids and some fats, proteins and carbohydrates, and must be combined with some B-vitamins in the body before the latter can be active.

Phosphorus is present in nearly all foods (Table 12). Furthermore, phosphates are added to a number of processed foods. High intakes of phosphorus in the first few days of life, resulting from the use of unmodified cow's milk, may produce low levels of calcium in the blood, and muscular spasms (tetany). This milk has a high ratio of phosphorus to calcium compared with human milk, and the calcium present in it may combine with the fat present and be poorly absorbed.

Most people should be able to get all the phosphorus they need by eating a varied and balanced diet. No additional intake is considered necessary for pregnancy, although an increase is recommended during lactation. In 2000-01 the average daily intake from food was about 1500 mg for men and 1100 mg for women, well above the Reference Nutrient Intake (p. 77). High intakes have been associated with mild gastrointestinal symptoms. However, guidance suggests that taking up to 250 mg of phosphorus a day in the form of supplements is unlikely to cause any adverse effects.

Table 12. Phosphorus and magnesium content of selected foods (edible portion)

	Phosphorus (mg/100 g)	Magnesium (mg/100 g)
Milk, semi skimmed	94	11
Cheese, Cheddar	505	29
Eggs, chicken, whole, boiled	200	12
Beef, stewing steak, stewed	180	19
Chicken, roast, meat only	200	23
Ham	340	24
Cod, fillets, baked	190	26
Sardines, in tomato sauce	420	39
Cabbage, boiled	25	4
Baked beans, reheated	100	31
Potatoes, old, boiled	31	14
Oranges	21	10
Peanuts, dry, roasted	420	190
Bread, white	95	23
Bread, wholemeal	202	66
Chapati, made without fat	120	37
Yeast extract	950	160

The main sources of phosphorus in the diet are cereals and cereal products (especially bread and breakfast cereals), milk and milk products (especially semi-skimmed milk), and meat and meat products. The main sources of magnesium are cereals and cereal products (especially bread and breakfast cereals), drinks (including beer and lager, coffee and tea), meat and meat products, milk and milk products, and potatoes and savoury snacks.

MAGNESIUM

Most of the magnesium in the body is present in the bones, but it is also an essential constituent of all cells and is necessary for the functioning of some of the enzymes that are involved in energy utilisation. It is thought that magnesium may help to lower high blood pressure. Magnesium is widespread in foods (see Table 12), especially those of vegetable origin because it is an essential constituent of chlorophyll. Less than half is normally absorbed and, unlike the chemically related element calcium, this process is unaffected by vitamin D. In 2000-01, food provided on average about 300 mg and about 230 mg magnesium per day for men and women, respectively. Deficiency is rare, and results from excessive losses in diarrhoea rather than from low intakes. No additional magnesium is required during pregnancy, but an extra 50 mg per day is needed during lactation to offset secretion in breast milk. Most people should be able to get all the magnesium they need by eating a varied and balanced diet. Guidance suggests that people are unlikely to experience adverse effects if they take 400 mg or less a day of magnesium in the form of supplements.

SODIUM AND CHLORIDE

Functions

Sodium and chloride are found in those body fluids outside the cells, such as blood. They are both essential in small amounts in the diet for maintaining the water balance of the body, and for muscle and nerve activity.

Absorption and excretion

The concentrations of sodium and chloride in the body are maintained within close limits and are controlled by the kidneys, through excretion and conservation. The ability of the kidneys to regulate the body's sodium content is dependent on a number of factors, including age. For example, older adults and very young infants cannot tolerate high sodium intakes because their kidneys cannot excrete the excess.

Sources and intakes

Sodium and chloride are added to the diet as salt, which is the main source of sodium in the diet. Habitually high salt intakes have been associated with high blood pressure, also called hypertension, which can increase the risk of stroke and heart disease. The evidence for the association between salt and blood pressure relates to sodium.

Some additives used in food (e.g. the flavour enhancer monosodium glutamate) contain sodium, but these make a comparatively small contribution to intakes. The main categories of food that contribute to sodium intakes in Britain are bread and meat products. Table 13 shows the amounts of sodium in selected foods. The sodium content of all foods that have not been processed is comparatively low, but salt is added to many prepared foods. The salt added during cooking or at the table, and the salt found naturally in most foods, makes up only a quarter of the salt in our diets. The rest (75%) comes from processed foods. For example salt is low in pork and other meats, but high in bacon, sausages and other meat products; low in herrings, but high in kippers. Foods where some products will be high in salt include soups, sauces, ready prepared meals, some breakfast cereals, pizzas, baked beans and savoury snack foods (e.g. crisps, nuts).

The average daily adult sodium intake in 2005-06, as estimated by measuring sodium excreted in the urine, was about 4.1 g for men and about 3.0 g for women, equivalent to about 10.2 g and 7.6 g of salt per day, respectively. This method of indirectly estimating sodium intake is used because it is not possible to measure intake directly since the amount of salt added to food in cooking or at the table cannot be accurately assessed.

In May 2003, the Scientific Advisory Committee on Nutrition (see footnote p. 10) made recommendations on the amounts of salt that the population should be eating. In order to help lower the average blood pressure of the population, and so decrease the prevalence of coronary heart disease and stroke, current recommendations are that the average sodium intake of the adult population should not exceed 2.4 g sodium (6 g salt) per day. In 2000-01, 85% of men and 69% of women had salt intakes greater than this. The recommended maximum intake of 6 g per day is higher than the RNI (p. 78) and substantially greater than the salt intake needed to maintain the sodium content of the body in a temperate climate. This amount is not an optimal level of salt intake but is considered an achievable population goal. Children under 11 years should be having less than this.

The maximum amount of salt babies and children should be having varies by age:

- Up to 6 months old – less than 1 g a day
- 7 to 12 months – 1 g a day
- 1 to 3 years – 2 g a day
- 4 to 6 years – 3 g a day
- 7 to 10 years – 5 g a day

Babies who are breast-fed receive the right amount of sodium through breast milk, and infant formula is manufactured to contain a similar amount. Babies should not be given processed foods, such as breakfast cereals and pasta sauces, which are not made specifically for them because these can be high in salt.

There is currently no reliable estimate of the amount of salt consumed by children, but available information suggests that it is substantially higher than these targets. From the age of 11, children should be having no more than about 6 g a day. This is the same level that is recommended for adults.

The UK Government considers salt reduction to be a priority for public health action and has set a target to reduce the average salt intake of the population to 6g per person per day by 2010 through public campaigning and working with the food industry to reduce levels in processed foods. In 2005 evidence suggested that consumers were already cutting down on salt. The Government is also working to set targets for levels of salt in a wide range of food categories with the aim of these being achieved by 2010.

Table 13. Sodium and potassium content of selected foods as bought (edible portion)

	Sodium (mg/100 g)	Potassium (mg/100 g)
Milk, semi-skimmed	43	156
Cheese, Cheddar	723	75
Eggs, whole, raw or boiled	140	130
Beef, mince, raw	80	260
Corned beef, canned	860	140
Bacon, streaky, grilled	1680	330
Sausages, pork, grilled	1080	190
Ham	1200	340
Chicken, meat, average, raw	77	380
Haddock, fresh, raw	67	360
Haddock, smoked, steamed	990	440
Butter, unsalted	9	27
Butter, salted	606	27
Margarine, soft, not polyunsaturated	880	5
Fat spread, (40% fat) not polyunsaturated	650	110
Potatoes, old, raw	7	360
Potato crisps	800^a	1060
Cauliflower, boiled unsalted	4	120
Baked beans, reheated	530	310
Baked beans, reduced salt	330	270
Peanuts, dry roasted	790	730
Tomatoes, raw	9	250
Bananas	1	400
Peaches, canned in juice	12	170
Raisins	60	1020
Bread, white	461	137
Bread, wholemeal	487	253
Cornflakes	1000	90
Muesli, no added sugar	47	530
Tomato soup, cream of, canned	400	190
Yeast extract	4300	2100
Soy sauce	7120	180
Gravy instant granules	6330	150

^{a} Average of values ranging from 600mg to 1500mg per 100g
The sodium content of vegetables is much higher if they are cooked in salted water. Apart from this, the main sources of sodium in the UK diet are cereals and cereal products, especially white bread and breakfast cereals, meat products including bacon and ham, milk and milk products, and food such as soups, sauces and condiments. The main sources of potassium are potatoes and savoury snacks, meat and meat products, milk, cereal products, vegetables and various drinks. Fruit and fruit juices are also noteworthy as being much richer in potassium than sodium.

POTASSIUM

Function, and effects of deficiency

Potassium is present largely in the fluids within the body cells where its concentration is carefully controlled. The total amount in the body is closely related to the amount of lean tissue. Potassium has a complementary action with sodium in the functioning of cells.

As potassium is found so widely in foods, deficiency is unlikely to occur. Like sodium, most of the potassium in the diet is absorbed and the excess is excreted through the kidneys. Losses may be large if diuretics or purgatives are frequently taken, and in cases of protein-energy malnutrition *(kwashiorkor)* where tissue breakdown as well as diarrhoea occurs. Potassium is essential to the correct functioning of heart muscle and in severe cases of potassium depletion, heart failure may result unless supplements are given.

Potassium, as well as calcium and magnesium, has been shown to have beneficial effects on reducing blood pressure. There is consistent evidence regarding the benefits of fruits and vegetables, which are a rich source of these minerals, on lowering blood pressure.

Sources and intakes

Potassium is widespread in foods, but is particularly abundant in potatoes, vegetables, fruit (especially bananas) and juices (Table 13). Most people should be able to get all the potassium they need by eating a varied and balanced diet. The average daily adult intake of potassium from foods in 2000-01 was about 3 g. Guidance suggests that taking up to 3700 mg of potassium in the form of supplements a day is unlikely to be harmful. However, older people may be more at risk. This is because as people get older the kidneys may become less able to remove potassium from the blood. Therefore older people should not take potassium supplements except on medical advice.

Trace elements

Though essential nutrients that the body requires in order to function properly, trace elements are required in much smaller amounts than vitamins and minerals. Trace elements are found in small amounts in a variety of foods such as meat, fish, cereals, milk and dairy foods, vegetables and nuts.

ZINC

Zinc helps with the healing of wounds, and is also associated with the activity of a wide variety of enzymes; about one-third of the comparatively large amount which is present in the body is in the bones. Zinc is present in a wide range of foods, particularly in association with protein, and meat and dairy products are excellent sources. About one-third of the zinc in the diet as a whole is absorbed, but this is reduced if large amounts of wholegrain cereals rich in dietary fibre and phytic acid are eaten, although the amount of zinc present in wholegrain cereals is enough to offset this. Average adult daily intakes from food sources in 2000-01 were about 10 mg for men and about 7 mg for women, which is adequate for most people. A small proportion (4%) of adults were below the Lower Reference Nutrient Intake (p. 77) for zinc. Most people should be able to get all the zinc they need by eating a varied and balanced diet. When supplements are taken, advice is that taking no more than 25 mg of zinc as supplements a day (the Safe Upper Level[1]) should not be harmful. If a higher dose is being taken under medical advice then this should be continued. High intakes from water stored in galvanised containers have caused toxicity.

The zinc content of selected foods is shown in Table 14.

Table 14. Zinc content of selected foods (edible portion)

	Zinc (mg/100 g)
Milk, semi-skimmed	0.4
Cheese, Cheddar	4.1
Beef, stewing steak, stewed	7.5
Chicken, roast, meat only	2.2
Ham	1.8
Pate, liver	2.8
Cod, fillets, baked	0.5
Eggs, whole, boiled	1.3
Potatoes, old, boiled	0.3
Bread, white	0.8
Bread, wholemeal	1.6
Chapati, made without fat	1.0

The main sources of zinc in the diet are meat and meat products, cereal products (especially white bread and breakfast cereals), milk and milk products (especially semi-skimmed milk and cheese).

COBALT

Cobalt is a trace element found widely in the environment. It can be utilised by humans only as part of vitamin B_{12} (p. 66). Good food sources of cobalt include fish, nuts, green leafy vegetables and cereals. Most people should be able to get all the cobalt they need from eating a varied and balanced diet. Average daily intakes from food are 0.012 mg per day[2]. Currently, cobalt is not used in supplements in the UK and intake levels from food are not harmful.

---

[1] The dose of a mineral or trace element that potentially susceptible people could safely take every day of their lives without medical supervision. In the case of those elements where there is not enough evidence to set a Safe Upper Level, Guidance levels have been set instead.

[2] Total Diet Study (TDS), 1994. The Total Diet Study is a model of the average diet in the UK. Foods representing the average diet, based on the Expenditure and Food Survey, (formerly the National Food Survey) are purchased from retail outlets across the UK, prepared and combined, for analysis, into 20 groups of similar foods. Analysis of TDS samples is used to estimate population average intakes of mineral elements and other dietary constituents.

COPPER

Copper is associated with a number of enzymes. Deficiency has occasionally been observed in malnourished infants, particularly if their initial stores were depleted by prolonged feeding of cow's milk alone (which contains less copper than most foods). Good sources include nuts, shellfish and offal (such as liver), but copper in the British diet mainly comes from cereal products, especially white bread, meat and meat products, potatoes, savoury snacks, drinks, fruit and nuts. The average daily intake of copper by British adults in 2000-01 was about 1.2 mg per day from food. Most people should be able to get all the copper they need by eating a varied and balanced diet. At the Safe Upper Level (see footnote p. 53) of 10 mg or less a day as a supplement, copper is unlikely to be harmful.

CHROMIUM

Chromium is involved in the utilisation of glucose. It is fairly widely distributed in foods; those with a high content include brewer's yeast, meat, wholegrain cereals, legumes and nuts. A safe and adequate intake for an adult is thought to be above 25 µg (0.025 mg) of chromium a day. Most people should be able to get all the chromium they need by eating a varied and balanced diet. The average daily intake from food is 0.1 mg[3]. At present, the Government advises against having any supplements that contain chromium picolinate because there is some evidence that this form of chromium could cause cancer. Research is being carried out to investigate this further. If chromium is taken as a supplement in other forms, guidance suggests that having 10 mg or less a day of chromium from food and supplements is unlikely to be harmful.

FLUORIDE

Fluoride is associated with the structure of bones and teeth, and increases the resistance of the latter to decay. Drinking water is an important source, but the natural content is variable and is often below the optimum level of 1 mg per litre (1 part per million). The only other important sources of fluoride in the diet are tea and seafood (especially fish whose bones are eaten). The use of a fluoridated toothpaste and mouthwash helps to prevent dental caries. It isn't clear how much fluoride is needed for good health. But it is known that people whose drinking water contains fluoride at about one part per million tend to have less tooth decay than similar groups of people where the concentrations of fluoride are much lower. In some parts of the UK fluoride is added to drinking water to improve dental health. Fluoride is not available as a food supplement.

IODINE

Iodine is an essential constituent of hormones produced by the thyroid gland in the neck, and most of the iodine in the body is in this gland. Deficiency causes it to enlarge - a condition known as *goitre*. The richest source of iodine is seafood. The amount of iodine in vegetable and cereal foods depends on the level in the

---

[3] Total Diet Study, 1997.

soil, and that in foods from animal sources depends on the level in their diet. Because of the widespread use of iodine in animal feed, milk and milk products are the main sources of iodine in the British diet, and alcoholic drinks such as beer and lager, cereals and cereal products and fish are also important. In countries with low levels of iodine in the soil, intakes are low leading to a high prevalence of goitre, and iodised table salt is beneficial. This is not an issue in the UK. Most people should be able to get all the iodine they need by eating a varied and balanced diet. The average adult intake in the UK from food sources in 2000-01 was about 186 µg per day (above the Reference Nutrient Intake (p. 77), with milk and milk products being the most important sources. Low average intakes of about 80 µg per day have been found in vegans. Edible seaweeds, which are rich in iodine, can be a useful source for vegans if used in moderation. Guidance suggests that having 500 µg (0.5 mg) or less a day of additional iodine in the form of supplements is unlikely to be harmful. However, excessive intakes of iodine can negatively affect thyroid function, which can lead to a wide range of adverse symptoms.

MANGANESE

Manganese is present in a number of enzymes and activates others. It is found in a variety of foods that includes bread, nuts, cereals and green vegetables (such as peas and runner beans). The principal sources in the British diet are cereals and cereal products, especially bread and breakfast cereals, vegetables (excluding potatoes) and drinks, particularly tea. Most people should be able to get all the manganese they need by eating a varied and balanced diet. Average daily adult intakes from food sources in 2000-01 were about 3 mg per day. Guidance suggests that taking 4 mg or less of manganese per day as a supplement is unlikely to cause any harm. For older people, taking 0.5 mg or less per day of manganese as a supplement is unlikely to cause any harm. This is a lower amount because older people may be more sensitive to manganese.

MOLYBDENUM

Molybdenum is found in a wide variety of foods. Those originating from plants that grow above ground – such as peas, leafy vegetables (including broccoli and spinach) and cauliflower – tend to be higher in molybdenum than roots or tubers that grow below the ground, or than meat. Foods particularly high in molybdenum include nuts, canned vegetables and cereals such as oats. Molybdenum is essential for the functioning of enzymes involved in DNA metabolism. Deficiency has not been reported in the UK and people should be able to get all the molybdenum needed by eating a varied and balanced diet. Average daily intakes from food are about 0.1 mg[4]. There is insufficient evidence about the safety or otherwise of molybdenum intakes above those from the diet, but the molybdenum intake from the UK diet is not likely to be harmful.

SELENIUM

Selenium is found in foods such as Brazil nuts, fish, meat, offal, eggs and cereals. It plays a key role in the control of thyroid hormone metabolism, immune function and in reproduction, and also helps protect cells by promoting the body's antioxidant defences. The dietary intake of selenium and the selenium status of the UK population have fallen by 30 - 50% over the past 20 years. It is thought that this decrease is probably related to the substitution of much of the selenium-rich high protein wheat for bread flour previously imported from North America, with lower selenium EU varieties of wheat, and to declining bread consumption. The average daily intake of selenium from food is about 40 µg[4]. The selenium status of the UK population, although not as low as that found in regions of the world that suffer severe selenium deficiency, may be marginal for the maintenance of good health.

In 1998, COMA[5] concluded that there was insufficient evidence relating current selenium intakes to adverse health effects. The issue may be reconsidered as more data become available. In the meantime, dietary advice on selenium remains that most people should be able to meet their selenium requirements by eating a varied and balanced diet. The Safe Upper Level for intake of selenium from supplements is 350 µg (0.35 mg).

---

[4] Total Diet Study, 1994.
[5] COMA was replaced by SACN in 2000 – see footnote p. 10.

8 Vitamins

Until the beginning of the 20th century, it was believed that the only components of a diet necessary for health, growth and reproduction were proteins, fats, carbohydrates and a number of inorganic elements. This view had to be changed when it was found that minute amounts of additional materials were also essential. These could be extracted from a variety of foods and appeared to be of two types: fat-soluble ('A') and water-soluble ('B'). They were later each discovered to contain several active components, or vitamins. The former are mainly associated with fatty foods and include vitamins A, D, E and K. The latter comprise the B vitamins and vitamin C. The vitamins of the B complex include thiamin (B_1), riboflavin (B_2), niacin (or nicotinic acid), folate, vitamin B_6, vitamin B_{12}, biotin and pantothenic acid. Vitamin C often occurs in different foods from the B-vitamins. Many of these vitamins exist in more than one chemical form.

The body needs fat-soluble vitamins every day. However this does not mean they have to be consumed every day as any quantity that the body doesn't need immediately is stored for future use. Water-soluble vitamins are not stored in the body, so they are needed more frequently. The absence of a vitamin from the diet or, more usually, its presence in insufficient amounts, leads to both general and specific symptoms. The most common general symptoms are, as with deficiencies of many other components of the diet, a feeling of malaise and, in the case of children, restriction in their growth. The specific symptoms of deficiency in humans are discussed separately for each vitamin. The amounts of selected vitamins needed to maintain the health of various age groups in the population are discussed in Chapter 9. Excessive intakes of most water-soluble vitamins are rapidly excreted in the urine. Because the body doesn't store water-soluble vitamins, these are generally not harmful. However, very high intakes of some, such as vitamin B_6 and niacin, can have adverse effects. Excessive intakes of fat-soluble vitamins accumulate in the body and can also be harmful. For example, high levels of preformed retinol (vitamin A) may have undesirable effects on the unborn child if consumed during pregnancy (see overleaf). The Expert Group on Vitamins and Minerals (EVM) has reported on the safety of intakes of vitamins used in food supplements and fortified foods (see reference in Appendix 9). The Group's advice or guidance for levels of vitamins taken as supplements each day that are unlikely to be harmful are given in each of the sections below.

Factors affecting the stability of vitamins in foods are discussed elsewhere (see p.92-93).

Vitamin A

The chemical name of vitamin A is *retinol* and it is found, pre-formed, only in foods of animal origin. Beta-carotene (ß-carotene – see p. 59) is found in foods of plant origin and can be converted to vitamin A in the body. The most convenient way of expressing the total vitamin A activity of a diet is as *retinol equivalents*: by convention, 1 µg retinol equivalent is equal to 1 µg retinol or 6 µg ß-carotene[1]. This average value takes into account the conversion losses and the lesser absorption of ß-carotene compared with retinol in the general diet.

Function, and effects of deficiency or excess

Vitamin A is essential for vision in dim light; thus prolonged deficiency (sufficient to deplete any stores in the liver, which in previously well-nourished people will last for 1 to 2 years) results in night blindness. In children in many parts of the world, deficiency also results in severe eye lesions (xerophthalmia) and complete blindness (keratomalacia). Vitamin A is also necessary for the maintenance of healthy skin and surface tissues, especially those that excrete mucus. Beta-carotene and other related compounds known as carotenoids, can act as antioxidants (see also p. 75), along with vitamins C, E and flavonoids and as components of fruit and vegetables are thought to have beneficial health effects.

Excessive doses, for example from taking large amounts of retinol (pre-formed vitamin A) preparations for long periods, accumulate in the liver and can be toxic. There is also an association between very high levels of retinol consumption during pregnancy and the incidence of some birth defects. As a matter of precaution therefore, women in the UK who are, or might become, pregnant are advised not to take vitamin A supplements, including fish liver oil supplements, except on the advice of their doctor and, as an additional precaution, not to eat liver or liver products since these can also be very rich sources of retinol.

Most people should be able to get all the vitamin A they need by eating a balanced diet. Some concern has been raised about the large amounts of vitamin A that some people get from their diet and/or from supplements. There is some inconclusive evidence that having large amounts of vitamin A over a long time may adversely affect bone health, making bones more liable to fracture. As a precaution, therefore, the Scientific Advisory Committee on Nutrition (see footnote p. 10) has advised consumers who eat liver once a week or more frequently, not to increase their intake or to take supplements containing retinol, including fish liver oils. They also advise post-menopausal women and older people at risk of osteoporosis not to consume more than 1500 µg (1.5 mg) of pre-formed vitamin A (i.e. not including ß-carotene) per day from diet and supplements combined. Guidance suggests that less than 1500 µg (1.5 mg) of vitamin A per day, is unlikely to be harmful.

---

[1] The amounts of vitamin A in foods are sometimes quoted in International Units (IU). To convert these to µg retinol equivalents, multiply the IU of retinol (in foods of animal origin) by 0.3, and divide the IU of beta-carotene (in foods of plant origin) by 10. (This is because I IU vitamin A = 0.3 µg retinol or 0.6 µg beta-carotene; and 1 µg retinol equivalent = 1 µg retinol or 6 µg beta-carotene).

Beta Carotene

The deep yellow or orange *carotenes* are responsible for the yellow or orange colours of many fruits and vegetables. They can be converted in the body to retinol and are therefore sources of vitamin A activity. Beta-carotene (ß–carotene) is the most important of them. The main food sources of ß-carotene are yellow and green (leafy) vegetables such as carrots, red peppers and spinach, and yellow fruits such as mango, papaya and apricots. Variable amounts of ß-carotene are found in carrots and dark green or yellow vegetables, roughly in proportion to the depth of their colour; thus dark plants such as spinach contain more than cabbage, and the dark outer leaves of a cabbage contain more than the pale inner heart.

Most people should be able to get all the ß-carotene they need by eating a varied and balanced diet. If ß-carotene supplements are taken, advice is to take not more than 7 mg per day of ß-carotene from supplements (the Safe Upper Level[2]) as more could be harmful. If a high dose is being taken as a result of medical advice, this should be continued. Beta-carotene supplements have been found to increase the risk of lung cancer developing in smokers and in people heavily exposed to asbestos at work. It is also possible that taking large amounts of ß-carotene supplements could increase the risk of cancer in other people. People who smoke or have been exposed to asbestos are advised not to take any ß-carotene supplements. There is no evidence to suggest that the ß-carotene intake from food is harmful.

Sources and intakes

Vitamin A is not widely distributed in food. Animals store vitamin A in their livers which are often extremely concentrated, but very variable, sources of retinol. Fish liver oils are also very rich sources of retinol. All margarine for retail sale is required by law to contain about the same amount of vitamin A as butter (see p. 111). This is now added to margarines and reduced fat spreads (although not by law for the latter) in the form of synthetic retinol and ß-carotene. Other good sources of vitamin A include cheese, eggs, oily fish (such as mackerel), milk and yogurt.

Average intakes of vitamin A (retinol equivalents) from food in 2000-01 were about 910 µg and 670 µg per day for men and women, respectively. The British diet as a whole provides well above the Reference Nutrient Intake (see p. 78) of this vitamin. However, a significant proportion of men and women aged 19 to 24 years had intakes from food below the Lower Reference Nutrient Intake (p. 77) On average women obtained about half and men two thirds of their vitamin A from retinol itself, with 21 per cent of overall vitamin A from liver alone. The amounts of vitamin A in selected foods are shown in Table 15. The main sources of vitamin A in the diet are meat and meat products, vegetables, milk and milk products and fat spreads. The contribution from liver and its products is higher in older people than in the younger age groups.

[2] The dose of a vitamin that potentially susceptible people could safely take every day of their lives without medical supervision. In the case of those vitamins where there is not enough evidence to set a Safe Upper Level, Guidance levels have been set instead.

Table 15. Vitamin A content of selected foods (edible portion)

Foods of animal origin	Retinol (µg/100g) only	Retinol equivalents (µg/100g)[a]
Milk, whole	33	36
Milk, semi-skimmed	19	21
Milk, skimmed	1	1
Cheese, Cheddar	364	388
Eggs, whole, boiled	190	190
Beef, stewing steak, stewed	0	1
Liver, lamb's, fried	(19700)[b]	(19710)[b]
Kidney, pig's, stewed	46	46
Cod, fillets, baked	2	2
Mackerel, smoked	31	31
Sardines, canned in oil, drained	7	7
Butter	958	1059[c]
Margarine, soft, not polyunsaturated	745	819[c]
Cod liver oil	18000	18000

	Carotene fractions[d]			
Foods of vegetable origin	Alpha-carotene (µg/100g)	Beta-carotene (µg/100g)	Beta-cryptoxanthin (µg/100g)	Retinol Equivalents (µg/100g)[e]
Sweetcorn, kernels, canned, re-heated, drained	0	22	180	18
Green beans, frozen, boiled	52	494	0	87
Lettuce, average of dark and light leaves	0	1020	0	171
Spinach, boiled	0	3820	39	640
Peas, fresh, boiled	7	245	0	41
Peas, frozen, boiled	26	558	0	95
Carrots, old, boiled	4170	11300	0	2230
Tomatoes, raw	0	564	0	94
Peppers, capsicum, red, raw	135	3170	1220	640
Peppers, capsicum, green, raw	9	260	0	44
Apricots, raw	2	405	0	68
Mango, raw	0	682	27	116
Bread		0		0
Potatoes, old boiled		0		0

The main sources of vitamin A in the diet are liver, vegetables (especially carrots), milk and milk products and butter and fat spreads.

[a] Retinol + (Beta-Carotene equivalents/6)
[b] Figures in brackets are estimated values
[c] Some types, which do not contain beta-carotene have lower levels than this
[d] The carotene content of many vegetables and fruit varies widely depending on variety and season.
[e] Beta-carotene/6 + Other carotenoids/12

B-vitamins

Although the chemical structure of each of the B-vitamins is quite different, they have several features in common. They act as 'co-factors' in different enzyme systems in the body. They tend to occur in the same foods and, being water-soluble, they are not stored for long in the body. These characteristics mean that diets containing too little of the B-vitamins can lead to *multiple* deficiency diseases within a few months.

THIAMIN (VITAMIN B₁)

Function, and effects of deficiency

Thiamin is necessary for the steady and continuous release of energy from carbohydrate. Thiamin requirements are thus related to the amount of carbohydrate, and more or less to the amount of energy, in the diet. The deficiency disease, beriberi, results from a diet which is not only poor in thiamin but also rich in carbohydrate, such as one based almost entirely on polished rice from which the thiamin-rich seed coat has been removed. In developed countries, most cases of thiamin deficiency are associated with alcoholism, where intake of the vitamin may be low and absorption and utilization impaired.

Sources and intakes

Thiamin is widely distributed in both animal and vegetable foods (Table 16). Good sources are pork, vegetables, milk, cheese, peas, fresh and dried fruit, eggs, wholegrain breads and some fortified breakfast cereals. It should, however, be noted that cooking may result in considerable losses from these foods (p. 92). Fats, sugars and alcoholic drinks contain no thiamin at all.

Wheat in the form of bread has long been a major source of carbohydrate in the British diet, but much of the thiamin is removed with the bran in the milling necessary to produce white bread. Thus a 30 g (about 1 oz) slice of wholemeal bread provides about 0.10 mg thiamin (0.37 mg per 1000 kJ; 0.16 mg per 100 kcal), while 30 g of unfortified white bread would provide only about 0.03 mg thiamin (0.1 mg per 1000 kJ; 0.04 mg per 100 kcal). It is therefore a legal requirement in the UK that all flour except wholemeal be fortified with thiamin to at least 0.24 mg per 100 g (equivalent to about 0.17 mg per 1000 kJ; 0.07 mg per 100 kcal see p. 104).

Most people should be able to get all the thiamin they need from a varied and balanced diet. In 2000-01 average intakes from food were 2 mg and 1.5 mg per day for men and women, respectively, well above average requirements.

Guidance suggests that having 100 mg or less of thiamin a day as supplements is unlikely to be harmful.

Table 16. Thiamin content of selected foods

	Thiamin (mg/100 g)	Thiamin (mg/1000 kJ)
Milk, semi skimmed	0.04	0.21
Bacon, streaky, fried	0.75	0.54
Beef, stewing steak, stewed	0.03	0.04
Corned beef, canned	0.00	0.00
Ham	0.80	1.77
Chicken, roast, meat only	0.07	0.09
Pork chop, grilled, lean	0.78	1.01
Sausage, pork, grilled	0.00	0.00
Sugar	0.00	0.00
Peas, frozen, boiled	0.26	0.89
Potatoes, old, boiled	0.18	0.59
Lentils, red, boiled	0.11	0.26
Oranges	0.11	0.70
Pineapple, canned in juice	0.09	0.45
Peanuts, dry roasted	0.18	0.07
Bread, white, average	0.24	0.26
Bread, wholemeal, average	0.25	0.27
Chapati, made without fat	0.23	0.27
Cornflakes, fortified	1.20	0.75
Rice, easy cook, white, boiled	0.01	0.02
Rice, brown, boiled	0.14	0.24
Spaghetti, white, boiled	0.01	0.02
Spaghetti, wholemeal, boiled	0.21	0.43
Yeast extract	4.10	5.37
Lager	0.00	0.00

The main sources of thiamin in the diet are cereals and cereal products (especially fortified breakfast cereals and white bread), meat and meat products (especially bacon and ham), vegetables, and potatoes and savoury snacks.

RIBOFLAVIN (VITAMIN B$_2$)

Function, and effects of deficiency

Riboflavin is a bright yellow substance, which is essential for the utilisation of energy from food. Specific deficiency signs are rarely seen in humans, but include sores in the corners of the mouth.

Sources and intakes

Riboflavin is found in small amounts in many foods (Table 17). Good sources include milk, eggs, fortified breakfast cereals, rice and mushrooms. About one third of the average intake in Britain is derived from one source alone - milk and its products. UV light can destroy riboflavin, so ideally these foods should be kept out of direct sunlight (e.g. bottled milk should not be allowed to stay too long on the doorstep). Some people in the UK, such as vegans, who avoid milk, have low intakes.

Table 17. Riboflavin content of selected foods (edible portion)

	Riboflavin (mg/100 g)
Milk, semi-skimmed	0.24
Cheese, Cheddar	0.39
Beef, stewing steak, stewed	0.15
Chicken, roast, meat only	0.11
Liver, lamb's, fried	5.65
Kidney, pig's, stewed	2.10
Eggs, whole, boiled	0.35
Red kidney beans, canned, reheated, drained	0.06
Potatoes, old, boiled	0.01
Brussels sprouts, boiled	0.09
Mushrooms, fried	0.34
Banana	0.06
Apricots, ready-to-eat	0.16
Rice, white, boiled	0.00
Bread, white	0.08
Cornflakes, fortified	1.30
Yeast extract	11.90

The main sources of riboflavin in the diet are milk and milk products (especially semi-skimmed milk), fortified breakfast cereals, meat and meat products and drinks (especially beer and lager).

Most people should be able to get all the riboflavin they need by eating a varied and balanced diet. In 2000-01, average intakes from food were about 2.1 mg and 1.6 mg per day for men and women, respectively, well above the Reference Nutrient Intake (see p. 77), although a significant proportion of women aged 19 to 34 years had intakes below the Lower Reference Nutrient Intake (p. 77). There is little evidence of any harmful effects of taking high doses of riboflavin supplements. Guidance suggests that taking 40 mg or less of riboflavin per day as supplements is unlikely to be harmful.

NIACIN

Function, and effects of deficiency

Nicotinic acid and nicotinamide are two forms of another B-vitamin (known collectively as niacin), which is involved in the utilisation of food energy. Both forms are found in food. It is therefore convenient to express the niacin content of foods in terms of equivalents: on average, 1 mg of niacin equivalent equals I mg of available niacin or 60 mg of tryptophan, and this is accepted as a definition. The amounts of both forms in selected foods are shown in Table 18.

Deficiency results in pellagra, in which the skin becomes dark and scaly especially where it is exposed to light. There are two apparent anomalies associated with pellagra: it occurs when the diet consists largely of maize, a cereal which contains nicotinic acid; and it can be cured by milk or eggs which are not rich sources of this vitamin. The reasons for these anomalies are firstly, that the nicotinic acid in maize and other cereals is largely present in a bound form which is unavailable to humans (although it can be released by alkali as in the preparation of Mexican tortillas), and secondly, that proteins of milk and eggs are especially rich in tryptophan - an amino acid which can be converted to nicotinic acid in the body.

Sources and intakes

Good sources of niacin include beef, pork, wheat flour, maize flour, eggs and cows' milk. Most people should be able to get all the niacin they need by eating a varied and balanced diet. Average intakes in 2000-01 from food were about 45 mg and 31 mg per day for men and women, respectively, well above the Reference Nutrient Intake (see p. 77).

Pharmacological doses of nicotinic acid (but not nicotinamide) can cause flushing, itching and burning sensations of the skin and nausea and gastrointestinal disturbance. Although evidence of the effects of taking high doses of nicotinamide supplements is sparse, guidance suggests that taking 17 mg or less of nicotinic acid as supplements a day or taking 500 mg or less of nicotinamide as supplements a day is unlikely to be harmful.

Table 18. Niacin equivalents in selected foods (edible portion)

	Total niacin (mg/100 g)	Tryptophan (mg/100 g)	Niacin Equivalent[a] (mg/100 g)
Milk, semi skimmed	0.1	48	0.9
Cheese, Cheddar	0.1	408	6.9
Beef, stewing steak, stewed	2.4	372	8.6
Pork chop, grilled	9.1	372	15.3
Chicken, roast, meat only	6.2	318	11.5
Salmon, pink, canned	5.9	264	10.3
Eggs, whole, boiled	0.1	222	3.8
Baked beans	0.5	48	1.3
Peas, frozen, boiled	1.6	54	2.5
Potatoes, old, boiled	0.5	24	0.9
Bread, white[b]	1.6	120	3.6
Bread, wholemeal	3.8	138	6.1
Wheatgerm	4.5	318	9.8
Tea, infusion	0.2	12	0.4
Coffee, infusion	0.7	0	0.7

[a] Available niacin + (tryptophan / 60)
[b] White flour is fortified to at least 1.6 mg niacin per 100 g by law.
The main sources of niacin in the diet are meat and meat products, cereals and cereal products (especially fortified breakfast cereals), and drinks (especially beer and lager).

PYRIDOXINE (VITAMIN B$_6$)

Function, and effects of deficiency

Vitamin B$_6$, or pyridoxine, is involved in the metabolism of amino acids, including the conversion of tryptophan to niacin; the requirements are thus related to the protein content of the diet. The vitamin is also necessary for the formation of haemoglobin. Deficiency is rare in humans and there is no evidence that women who are pregnant or taking oral contraceptives have requirements greater than other adults.

Table 19. Vitamin B$_6$ content of selected foods (edible portion)

	Vitamin B$_6$ (mg/100 g)
Milk, semi skimmed	0.06
Beef, stewing steak, stewed	0.23
Chicken, roast, meat only	0.27
Turkey, roast, meat only	0.49
Tuna, canned in brine, drained	0.47
Baked beans	0.14
Cauliflower, boiled	0.15
Peas, frozen, boiled	0.09
Potatoes, old, boiled	0.33
Yam, boiled	0.12
Tomatoes, raw	0.14
Oranges	0.10
Banana	0.29
Raisins	0.25
Bread, white	0.08
Bread, wholemeal	0.11
Rice, white, boiled	0.07
Wheatgerm	3.30

The main sources of vitamin B$_6$ in the diet are cereals and cereal products (especially fortified breakfast cereals), meat and meat products (especially poultry), and potatoes (especially potato chips) and savoury snacks.

Sources and intakes

Vitamin B$_6$ deficiency is unusual in humans since the vitamin occurs widely in food, for example: chicken, fish, liver, kidney, pork, eggs, whole grain cereals (such as oatmeal, wheat germ and brown rice), soya beans, peanuts, and walnuts (Table 19). Microorganisms in the intestine synthesise the vitamin, and some of this may be available to the body.

Most people should be able to get all the B$_6$ they need from eating a varied and balanced diet. Average intakes from food in 2000-01 were 2.9 mg and 2.0 mg per day for men and women, respectively, well above the Reference Nutrient Intake (p. 78).

If B_6 supplements are taken it is important not to take too much as this could be harmful. Taking large amounts of vitamin B_6 (more than 2000 mg), or taking it for a long time, can lead to a loss of feeling in the arms and legs – known as peripheral neuropathy. Generally these symptons are reversible so once the supplements are stopped, the symptons usually disappear. However, in a few cases when people have taken large amounts of vitamin B_6 especially for more than a few months, the effect has been irreversible. Taking doses between 10 and 200 mg a day, for only short periods of time, might not cause any harm. But there is not enough evidence to say how long these doses can be taken safely. The Government advises against taking more than 10 mg of vitamin B_6 as supplements a day (see footnote on the Safe Upper Level – see p. 59). If people are taking a higher dose under medical advice then this dose should be continued.

VITAMIN B_{12}

Function, and effects of deficiency

Vitamin B_{12} is a mixture of several related compounds, all of which contain the trace element cobalt. Together with folate, it is needed by rapidly dividing cells such as those in the bone marrow which form blood cells.

Because vitamin B_{12} does not occur in foods of vegetable origin, deficiency may occur in vegans who do not consume meat, milk, eggs, or any special supplement. It more usually arises, however, in those few individuals whose gastric juice contains no 'intrinsic factor' (p. 36) and who therefore cannot absorb this vitamin. Deficiency leads to a characteristic (pernicious) anaemia and the degeneration of nerve cells and occurs most frequently in older people. If a B_{12} deficiency state occurs, taking supplements of folic acid can mask this fact. An early sympton of vitamin B_{12} deficiency is anaemia. Taking large amounts of folic acid treats the anaemia without treating the B_{12} deficiency. If vitamin B_{12} deficiency is not diagnosed, it can eventually lead to damage of the nervous system (neurological damage). This is a concern particularly for older people, in whom vitamin B_{12} absorption can become more difficult.

Sources and intakes

Vitamin B_{12} occurs only in foods of animal origin, microorganisms including yeast and certain algae such as seaweed. Liver is the richest source, but useful amounts also occur in meat, fish, cheese, and some fortified breakfast cereals, as shown in Table 20.

If meat, fish or dairy foods are consumed then people should be able to get enough vitamin B_{12} from the diet. In 2000-01 average intakes from food were 6.5 µg and 4.8 µg per day for men and women, respectively. Adverse effects in humans are rare and there is little evidence to show what the effects might be of taking high doses of vitamin B_{12} supplements for long periods. Guidance suggests that taking 2 mg or less of vitamin B_{12} as supplements a day is unlikely to be harmful.

Table 20. Vitamin B_{12} content of selected foods (edible portion)

	Vitamin B_{12} ($\mu g / 100$ g)
Milk, whole	0.9
Milk, semi-skimmed	0.4
Cheese, Cheddar	2.4
Eggs, whole, boiled	1.1
Beef or lamb, mince, stewed	2
Pork chop, grilled	1
Liver, lamb's, fried	83
Pate, liver	8
Kipper, grilled	12.0
Cod, fillets, baked	2.0
Tuna, canned in brine, drained	4
Cornflakes, fortified	0.9
Yeast extract	1
Seaweed, nori, dried, raw	27.5
Seaweed, Wakame, dried, raw	2.5

The main sources of vitamin B_{12} in the diet are milk and milk products (especially semi-skimmed milk), meat and meat products (especially liver and liver products) and oily fish.

FOLATE

Function, and effects of deficiency

The term folate covers folates that are present in foods and the synthetic form, folic acid, which is not naturally present in significant amounts in foods. Folic acid is used for food fortification and in supplements. Folate has several functions, including its action with vitamin B_{12} in rapidly dividing cells. Deficiency leads to a characteristic (megaloblastic) form of anaemia, which must be distinguished from that caused by a deficiency of vitamin B_{12}. Folate deficiency can result not only from a poor diet, but also from increased needs for the synthesis of red blood cells in pregnant women, from increased requirements arising from certain medical conditions in the elderly and when there is decreased absorption of folate in gastro-intestinal disease.

Women who increase their folic acid/folate intake before pregnancy and during its early stages can help to reduce their risk of having a baby with a neural tube defect (NTD) such as anencephaly or spina bifida, in which the brain or spinal cord or their protective coverings fail to develop properly. To reduce the risk of an occurrence of NTD, all women planning a pregnancy are advised to take a daily dietary supplement of 0.4 mg folic acid and eat plenty of folate-rich foods prior to conception and up to the twelfth week of pregnancy. It is a good idea for all women of child bearing age to follow this advice if there is the potential for an unplanned pregnancy. To reduce the risk of recurrence of NTD, those who have already had an affected pregnancy should take a supplement of 4 or 5 mg folic acid daily before becoming pregnant and up to the twelfth week of pregnancy.

Sources and intakes

Folate occurs in small amounts in many foods. Good sources include green leafy vegetables (such as broccoli and Brussels sprouts), peas, chickpeas, yeast extract, brown rice and some fruit (such as oranges and bananas). Other useful sources include fortified breakfast cereals and some breads. Liver and its products are very rich sources but are not suitable for enhancing intakes by women who are, or might become, pregnant (see Vitamin A p. 58). Folate is readily destroyed in cooking, much being lost in the water used for cooking vegetables, and it is also readily oxidised to unavailable forms of the vitamin. Thus care should be taken to include several good sources of folate in the diet and to cook vegetables in only a little water for a short time to minimise the risk of deficiency. Selected sources of folate are shown in Table 21.

Apart from women planning a pregnancy, most people should be able to get all the folate they need by eating a varied and balanced diet. In 2000-01 average intakes from food were about 340 µg and 250 µg per day for men and women, respectively, which are above the Reference Nutrient Intake (p. 78).

Guidance suggests that taking 1 mg (1000 µg) or less of folic acid supplements a day is unlikely to be harmful.

See also folic acid and vitamin B_{12} on p. 67.

Table 21. Folate content of selected foods (edible portion)

	Folate (µg/100 g)
Cornflakes	333
Weetabix	170
Bread, wholemeal	40
Bread, white	25
Potatoes, old, boiled	19
Peas, frozen, boiled	47
Broccoli, boiled	64
Brussels sprouts, boiled	110
Lettuce	55
Okra, boiled	46
Apples, eating	1
Bananas	14
Oranges	31
Raisins	10
Almonds	48
Peanuts, plain, unsalted	110
Peanuts, dry roasted	44
Blackeye beans, boiled	210
Chickpeas, boiled	66
Egg, chicken, boiled	39
Kidney, ox, stewed	130
Beef, stewed	11
Cheese, Cheddar	31
Milk, semi-skimmed	6

The main sources of folate in the diet are cereals and cereal products (especially fortified breakfast cereals), vegetables, potatoes and savoury snacks, and drinks (especially beer and lager).

PANTOTHENIC ACID

Pantothenic acid is necessary for the release of energy from fat and carbohydrate. Dietary deficiencies of this vitamin are unlikely in humans because it is so widespread in food. Good sources include chicken, beef, potatoes, porridge, tomatoes, liver, kidney, yeast, eggs, broccoli and wholegrains such as brown rice and wholemeal bread. Breakfast cereals are also a good source if they have been fortified with pantothenic acid. Most people can get all the pantothenic acid they need by eating a varied and balanced diet. Average daily intakes from food in 2000-01 were about 7 mg for men and about 5 mg for women, which is within the range considered adequate. There is not enough evidence at present to know what the effects might be of taking high doses of pantothenic acid supplements for an extended period of time. Guidance suggests that taking a supplement of 200 mg or less of pantothenic acid a day is unlikely to be harmful.

BIOTIN

Biotin is essential for the metabolism of fat. Very small amounts are required, and sufficient may well be made by the bacteria normally inhabiting the large intestine. It is therefore probable that no additional biotin need be provided in the diet, except in the very unusual situation when large quantities of raw eggs are consumed[3]. Raw, but not cooked, egg white contains a substance (avidin), which combines with biotin making it unavailable to the body.

Biotin occurs naturally in a wide range of foods, but at very low levels compared to other water-soluble vitamins. Relatively good sources include meat such as kidney and liver, egg yolk, some vegetables and dried mixed fruit. Most people should be able to get the amount of biotin they need from a varied and balanced diet. Average daily intakes from food in 2000-01 were 41 µg and 29 µg for men and women, respectively, which are within the ranges considered safe and adequate. There is little evidence to establish the extent of risk associated with supplemental biotin. Guidance suggests that taking 0.9 mg or less of biotin as supplements a day is unlikely to be harmful.

Vitamin C (ascorbic acid)

Function, and effects of deficiency

Vitamin C is necessary for the maintenance of healthy connective tissue. It is a powerful anti-oxidant (p. 75) and is involved in preventing damage to the body by free radicals. It may also help to increase the body's absorption of non-haem iron (p. 44). Humans are among the few animals (along with monkeys and guinea pigs) unable to form their own vitamin C, and must therefore obtain it from food. Deficiency soon results in bleeding, especially from small blood vessels (capillaries) under the skin and from the gums, and wounds heal more slowly. Scurvy follows

---

[3] Older people, babies, toddlers, pregnant women or people who are already unwell should avoid eating eggs that haven't been cooked until the white and the yolk are solid, or any egg dish that has not been thoroughly cooked.

and, if the deficiency is prolonged, death results. Mild deficiencies may occur in infants who are given unsupplemented cow's milk, in people eating poor diets (for example some elderly people), and in people who have very restrictive diets that contain little besides whole-grain cereals which lack vitamin C.

Sources and intakes

Vitamin C is not widely distributed in foods. Small amounts occur in milk, especially breast milk, and liver, but virtually all the vitamin C in most diets is derived from vegetables, potatoes and fruit. Many people do not eat enough vegetables and fruit and vitamin C is readily lost from these foods during storage, preparation and cooking. Care should be taken to include good sources of the vitamin in the diet to minimise the risk of deficiency. The average vitamin C content of selected foods is shown in Table 22.

Citrus fruits and blackcurrants are particularly good sources, but some tropical fruits, such as guavas and West Indian cherries, are even richer. Synthetic vitamin C, which is equally valuable, may be added to fruit juices to compensate for losses during storage and to juice drinks which are only partially composed of fruit juice.

The amount of vitamin C in any particular fruit or vegetable may differ considerably from the value shown in the table. This is because of the natural variations which occur, the variable losses during the time between harvesting and consumption in the home, and the variations in cooking methods that may be used. As an example, fresh peas may contain between 10 and 30 mg per 100 g; the higher values would tend to occur in the spring and early summer when the plants are growing most rapidly, and may be preserved by freezing. The loss which can occur after harvesting is illustrated in Table 22 by the average change in vitamin C content of potatoes during storage; it can also be substantial in the days which elapse between the harvest of leafy vegetables and their consumption in the home. Vitamin C, like riboflavin, is also rapidly lost when milk is allowed to stand on the doorstep; this may be important for young children and those older people with restricted diets for whom milk may be one of the few sources of this vitamin.

Table 22. Vitamin C content of selected foods (edible portion)

	Raw (mg/100 g)	After boiling (mg/100 g)
Courgettes	21	11
Carrots, old	6	2
Cabbage, average	49	20
Cauliflower	43	27
Lettuce	5	
Pepper, green	120	69
Plantain (green banana)	15	9
Potatoes, new, average	16	15
Potatoes, old, freshly dug from	21	
stored 3 months	9	
stored 9 months	7	
average	11	6
Sweetpotato	23	17
Tomatoes	17	12 (canned)
Apples	6	
Bananas	11	
Blackcurrants	200	115 (stewed)
Grapefruit juice	31	
Kiwi fruit	59	
Mangoes	37	
Melon, cantaloupe	26	
Oranges	54	

The main sources of vitamin C in the diet are drinks in the form of fruit juices and soft drinks with added vitamin C, vegetables, fruit and potatoes. The vitamin C content of many vegetables and fruits varies widely, depending on variety, season and freshness.

The highest contributions to vitamin C intake in the UK are made by drinks in the form of fruit juices and soft drinks with added vitamin C, fruit and vegetables, and potatoes also contribute a significant amount as the large quantities eaten more than compensate for their comparatively modest content of this vitamin. The only vegetable materials containing no vitamin C are cereal grains (unless they are allowed to sprout) and dried peas and beans.

Most people should be able to get all the vitamin C they need from a varied and balanced diet. Average daily intakes from food in 2000-01 by men and women, respectively, were about 83 mg and 81 mg, well above the Reference Nutrient Intake (p. 78). Taking large doses (more than 1000 mg per day) can cause gastrointestinal disturbances. Since vitamin C may increase uptake of iron from the gut it is possible that high intakes may affect vulnerable people who suffer from conditions where they are unable to regulate iron absorption. However, guidance suggests that taking 1000 mg or less of vitamin C supplements a day is unlikely to cause any significant adverse effects.

Claims that extremely large amounts of vitamin C cure colds and other minor ailments have little scientific basis.

Vitamin D

Function, and effects of deficiency and excess

Vitamin D helps to maintain bone mineralisation by ensuring a plentiful supply of calcium in the blood. It achieves this primarily by enhancing the absorption of dietary calcium from the intestine, but it may also have a direct positive effect on the deposition of calcium in bone. Infants and children who are deprived of vitamin D develop rickets, with deformed bones which are too weak to support their weight. Because these changes readily become permanent, it is important to prevent their development; hence in the UK and some other countries, preparations containing vitamin D are available for children and pregnant women, and margarine and many reduced-fat spreads and milk products are fortified. Some adolescents and women who are repeatedly pregnant and who breastfeed all their babies, and some elderly people, may also suffer from bone softening (osteomalacia), resulting in skeletal pain and bone fractures, because they absorb too little calcium from a diet which is low in both calcium and vitamin D.

Sources and intakes

Vitamin D is obtained both from the action of sunlight on a substance in the skin, and from the diet. Sunlight is by far the most important source for most people, who will need little or no extra from food. But several groups of people should ensure that their food contains sufficient vitamin D: children and pregnant and lactating women, whose requirements are especially high, and those who receive little exposure to sunlight such as older housebound people or members of certain ethnic communities who prefer to wear enveloping clothes.

Few foods contain vitamin D. All those which do so naturally are products of animal origin, and contain vitamin D_3 (cholecalciferol) derived as in humans from the action of sunlight on the animal's skin or from its own food. There may thus be seasonal variations in the amounts present. Good sources are oily fish, liver, milk and eggs. Vitamin D_3 is also used to fortify a number of foods, as (sometimes) is vitamin D_2 (ergocalciferol), which appears to be equally effective in humans and can readily be manufactured using plant materials. Vitamin D is required by law to be added to margarine for retail sale (p. 111) and is also added to most reduced-fat spreads. It is also included in the supplements provided (free to those in need) in the UK to pregnant and lactating women and to children up to 5 years old. Table 23 shows some food sources of vitamin D.

Table 23. Vitamin D content of selected foods (edible portion)

	Vitamin D (µg/100 g)
Milk, whole	0.0
Milk, skimmed, dried, fortified	2.1
Evaporated milk, whole, fortified	4.0
Cheese, Cheddar	0.3
Eggs, whole, boiled	1.8
Stewing steak, stewed	0.6
Liver, lamb's, fried	0.9
Herring , grilled	16.1
Salmon, canned in brine, drained	9.2
Sardines, canned in tomato sauce	8.0
Tuna, canned in oil, drained	3.0
Butter	0.9
Margarine, soft, not polyunsaturated	7.8
Fat spread, 70% fat, not polyunsaturated	5.8
Vegetable oil	0.0
Cornflakes	0.0
Cod liver oil	210.0

The main sources of vitamin D in the diet are oily fish, meat and meat products, cereals and cereal products (especially breakfast cereals), fat spreads and eggs.

Most people should be able to get all the vitamin D they need by eating a varied and balanced diet and by getting some sun. Average daily intakes from food in 2000–01 were 3.7 µg and 2.8 µg for men and women, respectively.

The Government advises that pregnant or breastfeeding women should take 10 µg (0.01 mg) of vitamin D supplements each day. This is particularly if the women are of Asian origin, cover their skin when outside or rarely go outdoors. Older people should consider taking 10 µg (0.01 mg) of vitamin D each day, particularly if they rarely get outdoors or are housebound, always cover their skin when outside, or don't eat meat or oily fish.

Excessive intakes of vitamin D cause more calcium to be absorbed than can be excreted; the excess is then deposited in, and can damage, the kidneys, and can weaken bones. It is therefore necessary for vitamin D intakes to be carefully controlled, especially in young children. Guidance suggests that, for the general population, taking 0.025 mg (25 µg) or less per day of vitamin D as supplements is unlikely to cause adverse effects.

Vitamin E

Function, and effects of deficiency and excess

A number of related compounds (*tocopherols*) show vitamin E activity, the most potent being alpha-tocopherol[4]. Its major activity in the body is as an antioxidant. Vitamin E occurs widely in foods, mainly those of plant origin, and like other fat-soluble vitamins is stored in the body. For this reason deficiency is seen in only two groups of people. Premature infants who have very low fat stores develop an anaemia when fed on formulas low in vitamin E and rich in the polyunsaturated fatty acids which increase the need for this vitamin. Manufacturers now ensure, therefore, that infant formulas contain sufficient vitamin E. People who cannot absorb or utilise the vitamin can also be deficient.

Sources and intakes

Most foods contain vitamin E. Good sources are plant oils such as soya, corn and olive oil. Other good sources include nuts, seeds and wheatgerm (found in cereals and cereal products). Meat, poultry and dairy products also provide small amounts. The main sources of vitamin E in the diet are fat spreads, breakfast cereals, biscuits, buns, cakes and pastries, potato chips and savoury snacks fried in oil, vegetables and meat.

Average intakes of vitamin E from food in 2000-01 were about 10 mg and 8 mg for men and women, respectively, which are above what is considered adequate. Large doses of the vitamin may make the effects of vitamin K deficiency worse and hence affect blood coagulation (see below) and may cause a range of symptoms including headache and nausea. The Government advises that taking 800 IU (540 mg) or less of vitamin E from supplements each day (see footnote on the Safe Upper Level, p. 59) is unlikely to be harmful.

Vitamin K

Vitamin K is a group of compounds necessary for the normal clotting of blood. Deficiency can occur in a very few newborn babies so, to counteract this possibility, all babies should be given a supplement of vitamin K at birth. It also occurs in rare individuals who cannot absorb or utilise the vitamin. A dietary deficiency is unlikely, partly because the vitamin is widespread in vegetable foods such as spinach, cabbage and cauliflower, peas and cereals, and partly because certain bacteria present in the intestine can synthesise it. Guidance suggests that a daily supplement of 1 mg of vitamin K is unlikely to be harmful.

---

[4] Vitamin E activity is expressed as alpha-tocopherol equivalents. One International Unit (IU) of alpha-tocopherol is equivalent to 0.67 mg alpha-tocopherol.

Vitamins and antioxidant activity

Some carotenes, vitamin C and vitamin E are among the many substances in food that can have antioxidant properties. This attribute can help to counter the effects of reactive oxygen species (free radicals), which are produced by the body's normal metabolic processes. If free radicals accumulate they can damage key cellular molecules such as DNA and proteins. Cells which do not repair all the damage to DNA may be more prone to developing cancer. Free radicals can also readily oxidise polyunsaturated fatty acids in foods and in cell membranes in the body to give lipid peroxides which can also damage cells. Peroxides, for example those formed by the oxidation of LDL cholesterol (p. 17-18), may play a part in the formation of the 'plaque' which can build up on the walls of the arteries and eventually cause heart disease.

Experts have concluded that there is evidence that high intakes of fruit and vegetables are protective against some cancers. However, there is currently not enough evidence to identify any single component, or mixture of components, as being the active principle, nor that individual vitamins, for example in the form of dietary supplements (vitamin pills) protect against the development of cancers. There is also evidence that high levels of ß-carotene in the form of supplements can actually increase the risk of cancer in people such as smokers, who are at high risk. As well as vitamins, fruits and vegetables contain a wide range of other compounds with varying levels of antioxidant activity and it is possible that the range and mix of antioxidant vitamins and other compounds found in fruits and vegetables are necessary for effective protective activity. Research is continuing into the possible role of these compounds in the prevention of heart disease and cancer.

9 Dietary Reference Values for nutrients

An adequate intake of all the essential nutrients is needed for health and activity, and there are additional requirements for growth, pregnancy, lactation and in times of stress such as infection. The exact amounts needed are different for each individual, and depend not only on such readily quantifiable factors as height, weight and sex, but also on physical activity throughout the day, the rate of internal activities such as heartbeat, and the climate.

As these requirements can only be determined after lengthy experimentation, it is impracticable to determine them exactly for each individual. Instead, a number of national and international bodies have set standards in the form of recommended nutrient intakes for various groups of the population in question. These recommendations have generally been designed to ensure that the needs of most healthy people will be covered and are therefore higher than estimates of average requirements (except for energy and the energy yielding constituents). Conversely, the actual nutrient requirements of almost all individuals are less than recommended intakes. Therefore if a person's diet consistently contains more of a nutrient than is recommended, they are almost certainly obtaining more than their requirements. However, if it consistently contains less they could be wrongly diagnosed as deficient, although the further their habitual intake falls below the recommendations, the more likely they are to be malnourished to the extent that they show clinical symptoms. Recommended daily intakes (RDIs) or recommended daily amounts (RDAs) were useful for minimising the risk of dietary deficiency in a population, but they were often used wrongly to assess the adequacy of the diet of an individual when people did not understand how they were derived.

The *Dietary Reference Values* (DRVs), replaced RDAs in the UK in 1991. The DRVs cover a range of intakes for most nutrients and can therefore be used not only for assessing the adequacy of the diets of groups of people but also, in some circumstances, as a useful reference for those of healthy individuals in the UK. There are three values for most nutrients:

(a) the *Estimated Average Requirement* (EAR). An estimate of the average need for food energy or a nutrient. Many people will need more than this average and many will need less. The EARs for energy in the UK are shown in Table 24.

Table 24. Estimated Average Requirements for energy in the UK (per day)

Age range	Males		Females	
	MJ	kcal	MJ	kcal
0-3 months (formula fed)	2.28	545	2.16	515
4-6 months	2.89	690	2.69	645
7-9 months	3.44	825	3.20	765
10-12 months	3.85	920	3.61	865
1-3 years	5.15	1230	4.86	1165
4-6 years	7.16	1715	6.46	1545
7-10 years	8.24	1970	7.28	1740
11-14 years	9.27	2220	7.92	1845
15-18 years	11.51	2755	8.83	2110
19-50 years	10.60	2550	8.10	1940
51-59 years	10.60	2550	8.00	1900
60-64 years	9.93	2380	7.99	1900
65-74 years	9.71	2330	7.96	1900
75+ years	8.77	2100	7.61	1810
Pregnant			+0.80[a]	+200[a]
Lactating:				
1 month			+1.90	+450
2 months			+2.20	+530
3 months			+2.40	+570
4-6 months			+2.00	+480
>6 months			+1.00	+240

[a] Last trimester only.

b) the *Reference Nutrient Intake* (RNI), which is the amount of a nutrient that is enough for almost every individual, even those with high needs. The RNI is much higher than most people need and in practice it is very unlikely that anyone consuming this much will be deficient in that nutrient. The RNIs are broadly equivalent to the old RDAs. The RNIs for protein and selected vitamins and minerals are shown in Table 25.

(c) the *Lower Reference Nutrient Intake* (LRNI) is the amount of a nutrient considered to be sufficient only for the small number of individuals with low nutrient needs. Most individuals will need to consume more than this, and people who continually consume less will almost certainly become deficient in that nutrient. Since individual needs vary so widely, DRVs can only provide a guide to the adequacy or otherwise of a diet. Even when intakes are below the LRNI, biochemical measures of adequacy may be needed to determine whether there is really a problem.

Table 25. Reference Nutrient Intakes for selected nutrients for the UK (per day)

Age range	Protein (g)	Calcium (mg)	Iron (mg)	Sodium (mg)	Zinc (mg)	Vitamin A (µg)	Thiamin (mg)	Vitamin B₆ (mg)[a]	Folic acid (µg)	Vitamin C (mg)
0-3 months (formula fed)	12.5	525	1.7	210	4.0	350	0.2	0.2	50	25
4-6 months	12.7	525	4.3	280	4.0	350	0.2	0.2	50	25
7-9 months	13.7	525	7.8	320	5.0	350	0.2	0.3	50	25
10-12 months	14.9	525	7.8	350	5.0	350	0.3	0.4	50	25
1-3 years	14.5	350	6.9	500	5.0	400	0.5	0.7	70	30
4-6 years	19.7	450	6.1	700	6.5	500	0.7	0.9	100	30
7-10 years	28.3	550	8.7	1,200	7.0	500	0.7	1.0	150	30
Males										
11-14 years	42.1	1000	11.3	1,600	9.0	600	0.9	1.2	200	35
15-18 years	55.2	1000	11.3	1,600	9.5	700	1.1	1.5	200	40
19-50 years	55.5	700	8.7	1,600	9.5	700	1.0	1.4	200	40
50+ years	53.3	700	8.7	1,600	9.5	700	0.9	1.4	200	40
Females										
11-14 years	41.2	800	14.8[b]	1,600	9.0	600	0.7	1.0	200	35
15-18 years	45.0	800	14.8[b]	1,600	7.0	600	0.8	1.2	200	40
19-50 years	45.0	700	14.8[b]	1,600	7.0	600	0.8	1.2	200	40
50+ years	46.5	700	8.7	1,600	7.0	600	0.8	1.2	200	40
Pregnant	+6.0	[c]	[c]	[c]	[c]	+100	+0.1[d]	[c]	+100	+10
Lactating:										
0-4 months	+11.0	+550	[c]	[c]	+6.0	+350	+0.2	[c]	+60	+30
over 4 months	+8.0	+550	[c]	[c]	+2.5	+350	+0.2	[c]	+60	+30

[a] Based on protein providing 14.7 per cent of the EAR for energy.
[b] These RNIs will not meet the needs of approximately 10 per cent of women with the highest menstrual losses, who may need iron supplements.
[c] No increment.
[d] Last trimester only.

As well as those nutrients shown in Table 25, the Department of Health report[1] also gives DRVs for riboflavin, niacin, vitamin B_{12}, vitamin D, phosphorus, magnesium, potassium, chloride, copper, selenium and iodine.

A *safe intake*, in terms of the beneficial amount of a nutrient that would provide the needs of almost everyone, but below a level which would cause undesirable effects, was set for each of those nutrients where there was not enough information to estimate DRVs. These include pantothenic acid, biotin, vitamin E, vitamin K, manganese, molybdenum, chromium and fluoride. Further information on safety aspects in the form of advice and guidance on safe levels of higher intakes of vitamins and minerals, including those from both food and supplements, was published in 2003 (see Chapters 7 and 8, p.42 and 57).

There are also Dietary Reference Values for total fat, fatty acids, starch and sugars, and fibre (as non-starch polysaccharides - NSP). However, apart from certain fatty acids (see p. 12-19), none of these nutrients is essential, so that there is no actual requirement for them and EARs could not be set. Instead, desirable population average intakes were proposed for adults (see Table 26) with a view to improving health and reducing the incidence of diseases such as heart disease and cancer in the UK. The DRVs for fat, carbohydrate and NSP are not intended to be applied to children. Values have not been set for this group because research has not yet established the scientific basis for their needs. It should be noted, however, that children below the age of five, who need energy-dense diets, should not be restricted in their fat intakes.

Table 26. Dietary Reference Values for fat and carbohydrate for adults as percentage of daily energy intake

	Population average	
	Total energy[a]	Food energy
Saturated fatty acids	10	11
Polyunsaturated fatty acids	6	6.5
Monounsaturated fatty acids	12	13
Trans fatty acids	2	2
Total fat	33	35
Non-milk extrinsic sugars	10	11
Intrinsic and milk sugars, and starch	37	39
Total carbohydrate	47	50
Fibre as non-starch polysaccharides (g/day)	18	18

[a] Includes energy from alcohol

[1] Dietary Reference Values for Food Energy and Nutrients for the United Kingdom. Department of Health Report on Health and Social Subjects 41, 1991.

Energy

Appetite normally controls energy intake and keeps it close to requirements. However, this control is not perfect and energy intakes even slightly in excess of requirements are undesirable because they may eventually lead to obesity.

Intakes below requirements are also unsatisfactory. The recommendation for different sections (age and gender) of the population was therefore set at the EAR. Energy needs are calculated using basal metabolic rates (BMR - see Appendix 2) and physical activity levels (PAL - see p. 26).

$$EAR = BMR \times PAL$$

Although energy is needed during pregnancy for growth of the foetus, placenta and uterus, and for deposition in the mother's body of fat for use during lactation, there is also a reduction in physical activity and metabolic rate. Hence only a modest increase in the EAR for the last three months of pregnancy is recommended. Women who are underweight at the start of pregnancy may need to eat more than this. Energy is also needed for lactation, as breast milk contains enough energy to supply the needs of the growing infant.

Fat

Dietary Reference Values for fatty acids and total fat are given as their percentage contributions to energy intake (Table 26). These can be translated into quantities of fat or saturates per day for the average adult; 95 g and 70 g of fat per day and 30 g and 20 g of saturated fatty acids per day for men and women, respectively. These should be regarded only as guidelines to desirable intakes, rather than estimates of individual requirements, and are average values for the population consistent with good health. Apart from the essential fatty acids (see p. 14), there is no absolute need for these nutrients individually. A breakdown of the different types of fat (e.g. into saturated, unsaturated, etc.) has been included because their varying effects on health (p. 17-19) are as important to take into account as is total fat intake. The DRV for saturated fatty acids has been set with the intention of reducing the average blood cholesterol level of the population in order to help decrease the incidence of heart disease. To meet this target intake there needs to be a considerable change in people's diets; current recommendations are that present average intakes of saturates should be reduced from about 13 per cent to no more than about 11 per cent of food energy. It is recommended that average intakes of polyunsaturated fatty acids (PUFAs) do not increase. If monounsaturated fatty acid intakes also stay the same, or increase at the expense of PUFAs, total fat intakes must decrease to bring about a decreased intake of saturates. Average total fat intakes for the population are currently at the recommended level of about 35 per cent of dietary energy for the population as a whole. On average, adult women meet the recommendation for total fat, and men are close to meeting it, but a small proportion of the population still have fat intakes of nearly 50% of dietary energy.

Carbohydrates

Dietary Reference Values for carbohydrates are also given as their percentage contributions to energy intake. They are expressed in the following terms: non-milk extrinsic (NME) sugars; intrinsic and milk sugars and starch (for definition of terms, see p. 5-10). Non-milk extrinsic sugars are more detrimental to dental health than other forms of sugars, and it is currently recommended that the target population average intake be about 10 per cent of dietary energy (11% of food energy). Starch and intrinsic and milk sugars should therefore provide most of the 50 per cent of dietary energy to be derived from carbohydrate. As the present average intake of NME sugars is about 13% of food energy, many people will need to reduce their intakes of certain foods such as table sugar, confectionery, cakes, jam, honey and sugary soft drinks. In practice starch should always provide the major part of the energy intake from carbohydrate.

Average adult intakes of NSP should increase from the present level of about 14 g per day to about 18 g per day; more than 32 g daily has no extra benefit. Children should eat proportionately less. Small children under two years of age should not eat fibre-rich foods in place of other energy-rich foods or they may not be able to satisfy their energy needs. The amount of NSP in selected foods is shown in Table 2 (p. 11).

Protein

The DRVs are based on estimates of need. The protein RNI for adults aged 19 or over is 0.75 g per kg per day. Extra protein is allowed for growth in children, growth of the foetus and maternal tissue in pregnant women, and producing breast milk during lactation. The current average adult protein intake is about 17 per cent of food energy which is above the RNI but not likely to have an adverse effect on health. Since very high intakes will increase the rate at which kidney function is lost with age, it is recommended that protein intakes should not exceed twice the RNI.

Calcium and zinc

DRV's allow for the limited absorption of calcium and zinc from the diet and for the high needs of growing children and adolescents. There is no recommended increase in the intake of calcium for the period of pregnancy as calcium absorption is known to increase during this time, but extra may be needed during lactation to provide for milk production (see Table 25.)

Iron

DRV values allow for low absorption of iron, but assume that, in general, absorption is about 15 per cent from a mixed diet. Non-haem iron in diets containing no meat is not so well absorbed and habitual vegetarians may need higher iron intakes. The ingestion of foods rich in vitamin C at the same time as non-haem iron sources may help to improve iron absorption. The RNI for women of childbearing age is much higher than for other groups to take account of blood losses during menstruation, but women with very high menstrual blood losses may need intakes above the RNI. Such women may need to take an iron supplement.

Sodium

The RNI for adults of 1.6 g sodium (about 4 g of salt) is enough to satisfy the physiological needs of almost everyone and there is no advantage in exceeding this value. Habitually high intakes of sodium have been associated with high blood pressure. The present average adult intake of about 3.8 g sodium per day from food (equivalent to about 9.5 g of salt per day) is considered too high, and current recommendations are that the average adult population intake of sodium should not exceed 2.4 g (6 g of salt) per day to help decrease the incidence of stroke.

In 2003, the Scientific Advisory Committee on Nutrition (SACN) confirmed and strengthened recommendations on salt intake made by COMA[2] in 1994. They also made recommendations on the amounts of salt that babies and children should be having (see Table 25 and Chapter 7, p. 49-51). The target maximum salt intakes set for adults and children do not represent ideal or optimum consumption levels (they are above the RNIs), but are considered achievable population goals.

Niacin and vitamin A

DRVs allow for the contributions made by tryptophan and carotenes to the pre-formed nicotinic acid and retinol intakes respectively. Pregnant women should not take vitamin A supplements (except on medical advice) and should not eat liver or liver products, which are extremely rich sources of vitamin A. It is also advisable for post-menopausal women or older people at risk of osteoporosis not to consume more than 1.5 mg vitamin A per day from diet and supplements combined to avoid the increased risk of possible bone fractures (see p. 58).

Folate

The extra quantity of folate (or folic acid as a supplement) required by women who are or may become pregnant, in relation to reducing the risk of neural tube defects in their offspring, is described in Chapter 8, p. 67.

Vitamin C

Opinions differ about the quantity of vitamin C required for health. It is generally

---

[2] COMA was replaced by SACN in 2000.

agreed that 10 mg daily will not only prevent, but also cure, scurvy. The RNI of 40 mg for adults is thought to provide a reasonable safety margin. This is recommended to increase to 50 mg per day during pregnancy and to 70 mg per day during lactation. The evidence for possible benefits of significantly higher general intakes is still conflicting. (See p. 71 for guidance on high intakes).

Vitamin D

For most people in the UK the main source of vitamin D is from the action of sunlight on skin. There are therefore no DRVs for adults of the 18 - 65 age group. The RNI for people older than 65 years is 10 µg (0.01 mg) of vitamin D per day. Older people should therefore consider taking a supplement containing 10 µg of vitamin D each day if they rarely get outdoors, are housebound, always cover up their skin when outdoors or don't eat meat or oily fish. Supplementation to 10 µg per day for pregnant and lactating women and to 7 µg per day for infants and children up to 2 years is recommended to overcome seasonal depletion during winter months.

All children between six months and five years old could benefit from taking drops containing vitamins A, C and D, particularly if they aren't eating a varied diet, are of Asian, African or Middle Eastern origin or are living in northerly parts of the UK. Vitamin drops containing vitamins A, C and D are free for children from 6 months to four years of age in families on qualifying benefits through the Government's Healthy Start scheme[3]. They can also be bought cheaply from child health clinics.

Regulation of nutrient intakes

Excessive intakes of many of the minerals can be harmful, as can excessive intakes of some of the vitamins - especially vitamins A and D, which accumulate in the liver. Such intakes are unlikely to arise from food, but may result from the overenthusiastic use of dietary supplements (see also Chapter 8). Although our storage capacity for most nutrients apart from energy (as fat) is limited, the healthy body nevertheless contains enough reserves to last for many weeks or months even when few or no nutrients are consumed. Thus, while Dietary Reference Values are most conveniently expressed in daily terms, it is not necessary for the diet to contain these quantities *every* day. It is sufficient if the requirements are met *over a period of time*.

---

[3] Healthy Start replaced the Welfare Food Scheme in 2006. It covers the whole of the UK.

Uses of the Dietary Reference Values

ASSESSMENT OF DIETS OF GROUPS OF PEOPLE

For population groups, the EAR for energy and the population averages for fat, carbohydrates and fibre are used. If the average intake of protein, vitamins and minerals of the group is at or above the RNI, there will be very little risk of deficiency within the group. Conversely, the greater the percentage of the population below the RNI, the greater is the risk that insufficiencies or even deficiencies will occur.

ASSESSMENT OF AN INDIVIDUAL'S DIET

Since most estimates of an individual's nutrient intakes are not very accurate, great care needs to be taken in using DRVs for assessing the adequacy of the diet of an individual. An intake above the RNI is almost certainly adequate. Whether a person consuming an intake somewhere between the RNI and the LRNI is getting sufficient will depend on their level of need (high, medium or low), but the closer the intake is to the LRNI the more likely insufficiency becomes. However, because people's physiological needs vary considerably, deficiency of a nutrient cannot be diagnosed on the basis of dietary assessment alone.

PLANNING FOOD SUPPLIES FOR LARGE GROUPS

So that everyone in a group (for example in a school or older people's home) gets enough of every nutrient to satisfy their needs, those with high nutrient needs must be catered for. This should be achieved if the food supply provides the RNI.

NUTRITION LABELLING

Special nutrition labelling reference values that have been agreed across the EU are used for this purpose; the UK values do not apply.

PART 2

Nutritional value of food and diets

10   Introduction, and general effects of preparation and processing

Introduction

This part of the manual discusses the nutritional importance of particular foods in the context of the diet as a whole.

The nutritional importance of any food depends upon:

(a)   the composition of the raw food or ingredients as grown or purchased
(b)   the extent to which its nutrients are lost during storage, processing or cooking, and any addition of nutrients during manufacture
(c)   the amount that is usually eaten
(d)   each individual's own nutritional needs and the extent to which they have already been met by other foods in the diet.

Many factors combine to produce variations in the nutrient content of foods. *Representative* values for the most important nutrients in a wide selection of foods are given in tables throughout this manual and in Appendix 3, and these should constantly be referred to when using this part of the book. It must be remembered, however, that individual samples or brands may differ considerably from the values quoted here. A wider selection of foods and nutrients can be found in the book *The Composition of Foods (2002)*, and in its supplements as described in Appendix 9, p. 169-173, for those who wish to estimate nutrient intakes in more detail.

The general effects of storage, processing and cooking are discussed below, and the application of these principles to specific foods and menus is described in Chapters 11 and 12.

Average percentage contributions made by major types of food to energy and nutrient intakes from food consumed in Britain during 2000-01, and the average daily intakes of energy and these nutrients, are shown in Table 27. This table was derived from the National Diet and Nutrition Survey for adults aged 19 - 64 years, which included a nationally representative sample of about 1700 individuals aged 19 - 64 from private households across mainland Britain[1].

---

[1]   The National Diet and Nutrition Surveys constitute a programme of national surveys of various population groups with the aim of gathering information about the dietary habits and nutritional status of the British population. The results of these surveys are used to develop national nutrition policy and contribute to the evidence base for Government advice on healthy eating. Data from the adult survey has been used extensively throughout this Manual.

Table 27. Percentage contribution made by food groups to the nutrient content of the average adult diet in 2000-01

	Energy	Protein	Fat	Saturated Fatty Acids	Carbohydr
Cereals & Cereal Products	31	23	19	18	45
of which Bread	13	12	4	3	21
Breakfast cereals	3	3	1	1	7
Biscuits, buns, cakes & pastries	7	3	7	8	7
Milk & Milk Products	10	16	14	24	6
of which Semi-skimmed milk	5	6	3	5	2
Cheese	3	5	6	10	0
Eggs & Egg Dishes	2	3	4	3	0
Fat spreads	4	0	12	11	0
of which Butter	1	0	4	6	0
Meat, Meat Products and Dishes	15	36	23	22	5
of which Beef & Veal & Dishes	3	7	3	4	1
Chicken & Turkey & Dishes	3	12	4	3	1
Coated Chicken & Turkey	1	2	1	1	0
Liver, Liver Products & Dishes	0	0	0	0	0
Meat Pies & Pastries	2	2	4	4	1
Burgers, Kebabs & Sausages	2	2	4	4	1
Bacon & Ham	1	4	2	2	0
Fish & Fish Products & Dishes	3	7	3	2	1
Vegetables	4	5	4	2	4
Potatoes & Savoury Snacks	9	4	10	7	12
of which Potato Chips	4	2	5	3	4
Savoury Snacks	2	1	3	3	2
Nuts & Seeds	1	1	1	1	0
Sugar & Preserves & Confectionery	5	1	3	5	9
of which Chocolate Confectionery	2	1	3	5	2
Table Sugar	2	0	0	0	5
Drinks	10	2	0	1	10
of which Beer & Lager	4	1	0	0	2
Soft Drinks – non-diet	2	0	0	0	4
Fruit Juice	1	0	0	0	2
Miscellaneous	3	1	5	3	2
Average daily nutrient intake	8.38 MJ	75.3 g	73.5 g	27.8 g	273 g

Source: Food Standards Agency, National Diet and Nutrition Survey:
Adults 19-64 years, 2000-01
Figures have been rounded to the nearest final digit so there may be an apparent
slight discrepancy between the sum of the constituent items and the total shown.
*These values are for percentages from food and dietary supplements only. However,
average total daily sodium intake figure includes salt used in cooking and at the table.

NMES	Fibre (NSP)	Calcium	Iron	Sodium*	Vitamin C	Vitamin A	Folate
19	42	30	44	35	5	7	33
0	20	18	16	21	0	1	11
5	13	4	19	5	4	0	15
11	4	3	5	4	0	3	2
5	0	43	1	8	5	14	8
0	0	17	0	2	3	3	3
0	0	11	0	4	0	6	2
0	0	2	3	2	0	5	3
0	0	0	0	3	0	10	0
0	0	0	0	1	0	4	0
1	6	6	17	26	4	28	7
0	2	1	5	3	1	3	2
1	2	1	4	4	1	2	2
0	0	0	0	1	0	0	0
0	0	0	1	0	0	21	1
0	1	1	2	2	0	0	0
0	1	2	2	5	1	0	1
0	0	0	1	8	0	0	0
0	1	2	3	4	0	1	2
1	20	5	10	7	22	27	15
0	16	1	7	4	15	1	12
0	5	0	2	1	6	0	5
0	2	0	1	2	0	0	1
0	10	1	2	0	19	1	3
32	1	0	1	0	0	0	0
7	1	2	2	1	0	0	0
19	1	2	1	0	0	0	0
37	0	5	7	2	27	2	14
8	0	2	0	1	0	0	8
17	0	1	0	0	6	1	0
7	0	1	1	0	19	0	3
4	2	2	3	9	1	4	3
64 g	13.8 g	888 mg	11.5 mg	3.8 g	82.2 mg	787 mg	296 mg

Cooking and preservation

Most foods have to be prepared and cooked before they can be eaten. For some foods the process may be simple, as in the peeling of an orange. For others it may be complex: for example, wheat grains must be separated from the inedible parts of the plant and milled into flour, which in turn may need to be treated before being baked into bread. At each stage, some of the nutrients will be discarded or destroyed, whether the process takes place in a factory or in the home. The nutrients may be further reduced if the food is stored for long periods, particularly if conditions are not ideal.

Although these losses are usually not of major significance if a good mixed diet is eaten (as this will still provide a considerable excess of nutrients over the Reference Nutrient Intakes), it is nevertheless desirable that the losses are kept to a minimum. A discussion of the main methods of cooking and preserving foods is therefore followed by descriptions of the factors which tend to reduce the stability of each nutrient. Applications to specific foods are discussed in Chapter 11.

COOKING

Heat is generally applied to food in one of three ways:

(a) directly, with or without additional fat-as in roasting, grilling and baking (120-250°C; 250-475°F), and microwave cooking.
(b) with water - as in boiling, steaming, stewing and braising (100°C; 212°F).
(c) with fat -frying (155-225°C; 310-435°F).

Heat causes chemical and physical changes in food which in general make the flavour, palatability and digestibility of the raw product more acceptable and may improve its keeping quality. Heat may also increase the availability of some nutrients by destroying enzymes and anti-digestive factors. But cooking more usually results in the loss of nutrients, this being greatest at high temperatures with long cooking times, or if an excessive amount of liquid is used. The losses of soluble vitamins and minerals are, of course, reduced if meat juices and cooking water are not discarded but used in (for example) soups or gravies.

The effects of microwaves and infra-red cooking on nutrients are similar to the effects of the more traditional methods they replace. When used for reheating, they cause little additional destruction of nutrients.

FREEZING

This method of food preservation may result in some loss of thiamin and vitamin C when vegetables are blanched in water before freezing, but less than would otherwise result from the continuing action of enzymes in the plant tissues during storage. If the frozen foods are kept below -18°C (0°F) for a year there is little further loss of nutritional value until the food is thawed. In general, differences between the nutrient content of cooked fresh foods and cooked frozen foods as served on the plate are small.

INDUSTRIAL PROCESSING

Processing in a factory is mainly intended to preserve food so that the choice is greater and independent of geographical area or the season of the year, and to reduce the time spent on preparing food in the home. The main commercial processes which cause some loss of nutrients are blanching, heat processing, and drying or dehydration.

Blanching or scalding in water or steam is done mainly to minimise enzyme activity, and is a first step in the preservation of most vegetables for subsequent freezing, canning or dehydration. The process is usually carefully controlled, but small amounts of some minerals and water-soluble vitamins dissolve in the water or steam and are lost.

Freezing itself has little effect on nutritional value, and since the delay after harvesting is minimal the nutrients in the high-quality fresh foods that are used are generally well retained and can be present at a higher level than that of 'fresh' produce that has been stored for some time.

Heat processing in metal cans or bottling in glass jars will reduce the amounts of heat-sensitive vitamins, especially thiamin, folate and vitamin C. The losses will depend on the length of time needed to destroy any harmful organisms and to cook the food, and will be greater for larger cans and in foods of a solid consistency, such as ham, because of the slow transfer of heat from the outside to the centre. They will also depend on the acidity of the food and the presence of light and air, so that it is difficult to give precise values for expected losses.

Dehydration (in air) in carefully controlled conditions has little effect on most nutrients, but destroys about half the vitamin C. Thiamin is completely lost if sulphur dioxide is added as a preservative. Prolonged sun drying as in the production of raisins allows substantial changes to occur. Suitable packaging of dried foods is essential to prevent nutrient losses during their prolonged storage life.

High Pressure Processing (HPP) has emerged as a relatively new low temperature process, which destroys vegetative bacteria but has little effect on the sensory and nutritional quality of the product. Food products are subjected either in a batch or continuous process to a pressure of 4000 to 7000 times atmospheric pressure for around 10 minutes. There is a small temperature rise under the high pressure, and protein denaturation occurs. As bacterial spores may survive this process, products on the market processed by HPP have been restricted to acid foods such as fruit juices, smoothies, and dips. The process can be used to destroy pathogens in oysters and assist removal from the shell.

Stability of individual nutrients

PROTEIN

Protein is denatured by heat, and when cooking conditions are severe it becomes less available for utilisation within the body. This is partly because the changes in structure make the protein more difficult to digest and partly because some of the component amino acids are destroyed - most notably lysine, which can react with carbohydrates in the food. These losses can also occur during prolonged storage even at room temperature.

VITAMIN A

Both retinol and beta-carotene are stable throughout most cooking procedures, although there will be some loss at high temperatures and in the presence of air (e.g. when butter or margarine are used in frying or when vegetables are canned). Some loss also occurs during prolonged storage if light and air are not rigorously excluded.

B-VITAMINS

The *B-vitamins* are all water-soluble and most are also sensitive to heat.
Thiamin is one of the least stable of vitamins. It is readily dissolved out of foods into the cooking water and is easily lost in the juices from meat. It is fairly stable to heat if the food is acidic, but the losses can be considerable under alkaline conditions, especially if sodium bicarbonate is added during cooking. It has been calculated that on average about 20 per cent of the thiamin content of all the food brought into the home is lost during cooking and reheating, but the loss is greater in some foods than in others. Any foods that have been preserved by the use of sulphur dioxide, such as sausages and wine, will contain very little thiamin.
Riboflavin can be lost in discarded cooking water and meat juices; it is also unstable to alkali, and especially sensitive to light.
Niacin is an exceptionally stable vitamin, and will be lost only through its solubility in water.
Other B-vitamins are all soluble in water. Vitamin B_6, folate and pantothenic acid are also sensitive to heat, and can therefore be lost in cooking and canning.

VITAMIN C

Vitamin C is perhaps the least stable of all the vitamins. In addition to being water-soluble, it is very readily destroyed by air. This destruction is accelerated by heat, by alkali, and by the presence of certain metals, e.g. copper or iron. Vitamin C is also rapidly oxidised when an enzyme present in fruit and vegetables is released by any physical damage to the plant such as cutting. Thus poor cooking practices such as prolonged boiling of green vegetables in large amounts of water (especially if sodium bicarbonate has been added to improve the colour), followed by keeping them hot, can result in destruction of all the vitamin C originally present. Vitamin C is, however, partly protected by sulphur dioxide.

OTHER VITAMINS AND MINERALS

Vitamin D is stable to normal cooking procedures.

Vitamin E is not soluble in water and is stable to heat. It is, however, oxidised in the presence of air.

Minerals are unaffected by heat processing, but can be lost by leaching into water during moist cooking or processing.

Table 28 summarises the sensitivity of the most important nutrients.

Table 28. Summary of factors (✓) which may reduce the nutrients in food

Nutrient	Heat	Light	Air	Water	Acid	Alkali	Other
Protein	✓ if prolonged						
Minerals				✓			
Vitamin A	✓ with air		✓ with heat				Metals
Thiamin[a]	✓		✓	✓		✓	Sulphur dioxide
Riboflavin		✓		✓		✓	
Folate	✓		✓ (but protected by vitamin C)	✓		✓	
Vitamin C[a]	✓	✓	✓ (but protected by sulphur dioxide)	✓		✓	Enzymes; metals

[a] Least stable to cooking and storage.

11 Foods

Milk

IMPORTANCE IN THE DIET

Cow's milk is the most complete of all foods, containing nearly all the constituents of nutritional importance to humans; it is, however, comparatively deficient in iron and vitamins C and D. Unlike other foods of animal origin, milk contains a significant amount of carbohydrate, in the form of the disaccharide lactose (p. 6).

Typical amounts of the major nutrients present in 1 pint (568 ml) of whole milk and of skimmed and semi-skimmed milks are given in Table 29. Milk from the Jersey and Guernsey breeds of cow contains rather more fat than milk from other breeds (1 pint providing 26.7 g fat) as well as more beta-carotene and calcium.

Table 29. Nutrients per pint in various types of cow's milk[a]

	Whole	Semi-skimmed	Skimmed
Energy (kJ)	1605	1146	801
(kcal)	387	270	188
Protein (g)	19.3	20.0	20.0
Fat (g)	22.9	10.0	1.2
Carbohydrate (g)	26.4	27.6	25.9
Calcium (mg)	691	705	718
Iron (mg)	0.18	0.12	0.18
Sodium (mg)	252	253	259
Vitamin A (retinol equivalent) (µg)	213	120	6
Thiamin (mg)	0.18	0.24	0.18
Riboflavin (mg)	1.35	1.41	1.30
Niacin equivalent (mg)	4.7	5.3	4.7
Vitamin B_{12} (µg)	5.3	2.4	4.7
Vitamin C (mg)	12	6	6
Vitamin D (µg)	0	0	0

[a] To convert values to nutrients per litre multiply by 1.76
Values decline on storage in the home.

Average milk consumption is now just over one third of a pint (198 ml) per day, sixty per cent of which is reduced-fat milk (skimmed and semi-skimmed milk).

The contribution that these various types of milk make to the nutrient content of the average adult diet is shown in Table 27 (p. 88-89). It can be seen that in a mixed diet milk is particularly valuable for its content of high-quality protein and easily assimilated calcium; it is also a rich source of riboflavin. Moreover, milk provides good nutritional value for money.

Unmodified cow's milk is not suitable for infants under one year of age as their main drink because it doesn't contain enough iron and other nutrients. It is important that young children are given concentrated sources of energy. Thus whole milk, not reduced-fat milks, should be given to children between the ages of one and two years. Those over two but under five can be given semi-skimmed, but not skimmed milk provided they have a good appetite and are eating a varied diet. Semi-skimmed milk contains less fat than whole milk but has a similar content of protein and calcium. Skimmed milk does not contain enough calories for a child under five. Reduced-fat milks are, however, useful for adults who drink a lot of milk and who wish to reduce their fat intake (p. 16).

It is important that bottled milks are not left on the doorstep exposed directly to sunlight for more than an hour, since a substantial amount of the riboflavin and vitamin C can be destroyed.

EFFECTS OF COOKING

The bubbles of steam formed as milk is heated are stabilised by the protein and this gives rise to the characteristic 'boiling over'. Food such as fish or vegetables, when baked in the milk, can cause coagulation of milk proteins, but this does not affect their digestibility. Some caramelisation of the sugars in milk may occur with long cooking in a very slow oven, as for example in milk puddings or in the production of sterilised or evaporated milk.

EFFECTS OF PROCESSING

When milk is *homogenised* the fat globules are broken up mechanically and distributed throughout the milk so that they no longer rise to form a creamy layer at the top of the milk bottle. The nutritional value of homogenised milk is similar to that of pasteurised milk.

Skimmed milk has almost all of its fat removed, and *semi-skimmed milk* must by law contain only between 1.5 and 1.8 per cent fat. The fat-soluble vitamins A and D are reduced proportionately (only traces remain in skimmed milk), but the calcium content remains almost unchanged (see Table 29). *Dried skimmed milk,* and similar products with added vegetable fat, may be fortified with vitamins A and D.

A variety of heat treatments can be used to improve the keeping quality of liquid milk. The fat, fat-soluble vitamins, carbohydrates and minerals of milk are not affected by heat, but when the heat treatment is relatively harsh slight changes occur in the availability of some of the amino acids in the milk proteins. The vitamins in milk that are partially destroyed by heat processing are vitamin C, thiamin, pyridoxine, vitamin B_{12} and folate.

Most of the liquid milk supply in the UK is pasteurised by the High Temperature Short Time (HTST) method. During this relatively mild form of heat treatment the milk is heated to 72°C (162°F) for at least 15 seconds, killing any disease-causing bacteria. Between 0 and 10 per cent of the thiamin, riboflavin, vitamin B_{12} and folate, and about 10 percent of the vitamin C are destroyed, but in a varied diet, milk is not an important source of these nutrients. The ultra high temperature (UHT) treatment of milk, in which a temperature of at least 135°C (275°F) is maintained for at least two seconds, destroys all bacteria; it also causes some vitamin losses, which are similar to the losses in pasteurisation. UHT or 'long-life' milk is packed aseptically into special containers that protect it from light and from oxygen. It will keep satisfactorily for several months without refrigeration, but variable losses of vitamin C and folate (up to 50%) may occur during prolonged storage. Once opened, however, UHT milk is as perishable as fresh milk.

The old form of *sterilised* milk has been discontinued in the United Kingdom and most milk is now processed by either pasteurisation or UHT.

Evaporated milk is prepared by the concentration of liquid milk at low temperatures; the milk is subsequently sterilised in cans at, for example, 115°C (239°F) for 15 minutes. About 60 per cent of the vitamin C of the raw milk and 20 per cent of the thiamin are destroyed during the process.

Sweetened condensed milk is prepared similarly to evaporated milk, but since it contains added sucrose the processing temperature needed for an adequate storage life is lower. Nutrient losses are therefore lower too, and are generally similar to those that occur in pasteurisation.

Milk products

CHEESE

When rennet is added to warm acidified milk, the milk protein casein coagulates to form a firm curd which is treated in various ways to make cheeses of different kinds. Most of the protein, fat and vitamin A and much of the calcium in the milk remain in the curd, while a large part of the lactose and B-vitamins are lost with the whey as it drains away. Further minor changes in vitamin content occur during ripening and storage - processes that are greatly affected by the amount of salt present. Cheddar cheese consists very roughly of one-third protein, one-third fat and one-third water. Although methods of preparation differ, the amounts of protein and fat in whole-milk cheeses are fairly similar. Reduced-fat cheeses are also available. *Hard cheeses,* such as Cheddar and Double Gloucester, in general contain more nutrients per 100 g than *soft cheeses,* such as Camembert, because they contain less moisture. Some cheeses are not ripened, such as cottage cheese, cream cheese, fromage frais and quark. *Fromage frais* is a very soft cheese with a mild and fresh taste. Although its fat content varies according to the starting material, most products sold have a relatively low fat content compared to hard and soft cheeses. *Cottage cheese* is made from skimmed milk and therefore contains very little fat; *cream cheese* has a high fat content. Certain cheeses are made from milk other than cow's milk; for example *feta cheese* is traditionally made from goat's or sheep's milk and mozzarella from buffalo milk.

Pregnant women are advised not to eat soft mould-ripened cheeses such as Camembert, Brie or chevre (a type of goat's cheese) or blue-veined cheeses, due to the possible presence in these cheeses of harmful bacteria or viruses.

YOGURT

The nutritional value of yogurt is similar to that of the milk and minor ingredients used in its preparation, except that in products with added sugar or added fat the energy content is increased. Most commercial yogurts are based either on whole milk or on skimmed milk that is inoculated with a selected culture of lactic acid bacteria under controlled conditions. Dried skimmed milk, pectin or modified starch may be added to produce a firmer or more 'creamy' consistency; flavourings, fruit juices, fruit, nuts and sugar or non-sugar sweeteners are often incorporated to give a varied product. Some varieties of yogurt are fortified with vitamins A and D. There is also yogurt containing a constituent, made from plant extracts (*see Dairy Spreads* p. 111) that can help to lower blood cholesterol. Depending on the type of milk from which it is made, the fat content of yogurt can vary from about 0.2 g per 100 g in low-calorie yogurt to about 10 g per 100 g in Greek yogurt made with cow's milk.

ICE CREAM

The nutrient composition of dairy ice cream varies with the amounts of sugar, milk, dried milk, butterfat and cream that it contains. It can make a contribution to the daily intake of energy and calcium, particularly for people who have small appetites or who will not drink milk. Although most ice cream in the UK is based on skimmed milk with non-dairy fats instead of, or as well as milk fat, it is still a good source of calcium. Sorbets (water ices) are not based on milk, but consist of a mixture of water, fruit and variable amounts of added sugar.

BUTTER

Churning cream in a rotating drum so that the fat globules separate from the liquid buttermilk makes butter. In England and Wales butter must contain between 80 and 90 per cent milk fat, not more than 2 per cent milk solids other than fat and not more than 16 per cent water. During manufacture, 1-2 per cent of salt is added to salted butter. The amounts of vitamins A and D in butter vary; representative values are shown in Appendix 3. *Ghee* is made by the prolonged heating of butter. The emulsion breaks down and on cooling the pure fat can be separated from the water so that ghee contains virtually no water. Vegetable ghee, made from vegetable oil, can also be obtained.

CREAM

Cream is derived from fresh milk either by skimming off the fatty layer which rises to the surface or in a mechanical separator. Minimum fat contents for different types of cream are specified in Government Regulations; these include: half cream, 12 per cent by weight as milk fat; single cream, 18 per cent; whipping cream 35 per cent; double cream 48 per cent; and clotted cream, 55 per cent fat. These compare with an average of 3.9 per cent fat in whole milk. The energy value of different types of cream varies directly with the fat content. Sour cream is made by adding a bacterial culture to the cream to slightly sour it and give it a thicker consistency. Sour cream is nutritionally similar to the cream from which it is made.

Meat

The average nutrient composition of various types of meat is shown in Appendix 3. Genetic breeding and changes in methods of animal husbandry have resulted in leaner meat, particularly in the case of sheep and pigs, than that of twenty years ago. More of the external fat may also be trimmed off prior to sale.

Muscle tissue is composed of bundles of muscle fibres surrounded by connective tissue and associated with intramuscular fat. Each separate muscle fibre is a tube composed largely of water, and containing soluble proteins, mineral salts, vitamins and other components which give rise to flavours when meat is cooked. The eating quality of meat is largely determined by the relative proportions of connective tissue and muscle fibres in a particular cut and the amount of 'marbling' fat that is present within the lean, but the overall nutrient content of lean meat from the more expensive cuts is not significantly different from that in other parts of the carcase.

IMPORTANCE IN THE DIET

Meat is a good source of high-quality protein, of available iron and zinc, and of all the B-vitamins except folate. Pork, bacon and ham in particular are rich in thiamin. Liver and, to a lesser extent, kidney, are also rich in vitamin A and folate (thus differing from carcase meat) and in iron, riboflavin and other B-vitamins. Sweetbreads and tripe are useful and easily digestible sources of animal protein. Tripe also contains more calcium than other meats; this is derived from the lime with which it is treated during preparation. Liver and kidney and chicken and turkey meat (especially if the skin is removed) contain less fat than most carcase meat and their energy content is therefore lower. Much of the fat can nevertheless be trimmed from beef, lamb and pork before or after cooking. Mince may be heated and the melted fat poured off before further cooking takes place.

Consumption of poultry meat doubled between 1986-87 and 2000-01 and is greater than the consumption of beef. This trend is due to the growth of the broiler industry and the consequent fall in the price of poultry. Small differences in the nutrient composition of broiler chickens and free-range chickens are of no significance in a mixed diet. Recommendations for consumption levels of red and processed meat by adults are discussed in Chapter 3, p. 19.

Since there is an association between high intakes of retinol (vitamin A) during pregnancy and the incidence of some birth defects, women who are, or who might become, pregnant are advised not to eat liver or liver products, since these can be rich in retinol (see also under Fish, p. 100).

In addition, pregnant women are advised not to eat any type of paté or undercooked meat to avoid the possible presence of harmful bacteria or viruses.

EFFECTS OF COOKING

The muscle protein myoglobin which provides the red colour of raw meat is changed by heat, and the brown colour associated with cooked meat develops at temperatures above 65°C. Heat causes the proteins in the muscle fibres to coagulate and the meat becomes firm; shrinkage occurs and this in turn causes extrusion of meat juices and a loss of weight. Losses of fat and meat juices increase as the temperature rises, so the total weight loss is influenced by the cooking temperature and the internal temperature which the meat reaches as well as by the cooking time; thus the effects of grilling and frying are similar. The substantial variations that occur in the proportions of bone, muscle and fat in different parts of different carcases also affect the nutrients that are actually available from a given weight of fresh meat. It is thus very important, when estimating the contributions made by meat to the nutrient content of a diet, to weigh each cut after cooking and removal of any fat or bone.

Some cheaper cuts of meat which contain a higher proportion of connective tissue are more palatable if a slow moist method of cooking, such as stewing or braising, is used for the preparation; this allows the collagen in the connective tissue to be converted to gelatin thus making the meat more tender. Pressure-cooking is also useful for this purpose.

Cooking does not affect the minerals present in meat, but a proportion of those which are soluble pass into the exuded juices or dissolve in the cooking water. Similarly, since the B-vitamins are all water-soluble, varying amounts will be found in the drip, meat juice and stock. Losses of B-vitamins from fried or grilled meat are around 20 per cent. Destruction of thiamin, niacin, pyridoxine and pantothenic acid in stewed meat varies between 30 and 70 per cent, although overall losses are smaller if the gravy or liquid from a stew is consumed. About 30 per cent of the folate is lost from stewed liver and kidney. After cooking, there are only small differences in the content of the B-vitamins in fresh and frozen meat. Vitamin A is relatively stable to heat, and is not affected by most cooking procedures, although some loss occurs during frying at high temperatures (above 200°C).

There is no evidence of any significant loss of nutrients from meat during freezing, but the drip which collects on thawing will contain some soluble nutrients.

Meat juices are water-soluble substances from meat that include peptides, B-vitamins and mineral salts. They provide, with fat, most of the flavour and aroma of meat and act as a stimulant to appetite and to the secretion of gastric juice.

Stock can be made by boiling meat bones in water. The hot water extracts a small amount of fat and gelatin from the bone marrow together with other minor components that provide the flavour. Stock is usually used as a basis for soup and it is the addition of other ingredients (e.g. milk, fat and flour in cream soups) which provides most of the nutritional value of the soup.

Meat products

The meat content of meat products such as sausages is controlled by Government Regulations (see Appendix 8, p. 167). The important contribution that meat products make to the nutrient content of the average adult diet is shown in Table 27, p. 88-89; average consumption per head is rather greater than for carcase meat.

The most usual methods of heat treatment which meat products undergo during manufacture before any further cooking in the home are roasting, baking and canning, all of which cause some loss of thiamin and a slight reduction in the quality of the meat protein. The loss of thiamin when meat is canned is generally slightly greater than in cooked meat. Corned beef is prepared from cured meat which is trimmed, coarsely cut and cooked before canning; after this process very little thiamin remains in the finished product. Commercial *meat extract* is a by-product of the meat industry. The liquid in which meat and bone have been heated is concentrated after the removal of some of the fat. Such products, including stock cubes, are also rich in sodium. When the meat extract containing the dissolved solids is diluted again for consumption, the amount of protein and energy that it contributes to the soup or beverage is too small to be of importance in the diet; nevertheless it contains minerals besides the salt and vitamins, and is a useful stimulant to appetite.

The nutrient losses that occur during the cooking of meat products are similar to those that occur during the cooking of carcase meat.

Fish

IMPORTANCE IN THE DIET

The flesh or muscle of fish is a valuable source of protein, which is of a similar quality to that of meat and milk. It can be seen from Appendix 3 that the average content of fat in different kinds of fish varies widely; the flesh of white fish, such as cod, haddock, plaice and whiting, contains very little fat (1-2 per cent). In contrast, that of oily fish, such as herring, kippers (which are herrings that have been salted and smoked), mackerel, trout, salmon, and fresh tuna, varies from about 5 per cent to about 20 per cent. There can also be considerable variation within one type of oily fish, depending on the season of the year or the level of maturity attained by the fish. In general, the vitamin content of white fish muscle is similar to that of lean meat. The fat-soluble vitamins A and D are present in the flesh of oily fish and in the livers of fish such as cod and halibut. Oils from the latter may therefore be used as concentrated vitamin supplements. However, pregnant women should avoid taking supplements containing fish liver oils since these contain high levels of vitamin A which have been linked with birth defects. Fish oils also contain long-chain omega-3 polyunsaturated fatty acids that can help to prevent coronary heart disease (see p. 14) by decreasing the tendency of the blood to clot and reducing inflammation. For this reason, the Government recommends that people should eat at least two portions of fish each week, one portion of which should be oily fish such as sardines, mackerel or salmon. Taking fish oil capsules can also help protect against heart disease, but it is preferable to eat fish because it is an excellent source of other nutrients.

Fish muscle contains a well balanced supply of minerals including iodine, and if the bones are eaten, as for example in sardines and canned salmon, these are a good source of calcium, phosphorus and fluoride.

Pregnant or breastfeeding women and women who are planning a pregnancy have been advised by the Government to limit their consumption of tuna to no more than 4 medium-sized cans (drained weight 140 g per can) or 2 fresh tuna steaks per week (weighing 140 g cooked or 170 g raw), and to avoid eating shark, swordfish or marlin. Children under 16 have also been advised to avoid shark, swordfish and marlin. This is because these types of fish can contain relatively high levels of mercury. It is also advisable for pregnant women to avoid having more than 2 portions of oily fish such as mackerel or herring each week since these types of fish contain pollutants such as dioxins. There is no problem with eating other types of fish such as cod, haddock, plaice or salmon during pregnancy as part of a healthy diet. Other consumers have been advised to limit shark, swordfish or marlin to one portion per week, but do not need to limit tuna consumption.

EFFECTS OF COOKING AND PROCESSING

The changes that occur when fish is cooked are similar to those in meat but the shrinkage is not so great; losses of mineral salts are proportional to the loss of water. The vitamin A and vitamin D in oily fish are both heat-stable. Canned tuna is a poor source of the long-chain omega-3 polyunsaturated fatty acids (p. 16) as processing reduces the fat content of the fish to a low level. Canning of other oily fish has little effect on their fat content, so that canned sardines, pilchards, mackerel and salmon remain good sources of omega-3 polyunsaturated fatty acids. When fish is canned or cured by smoking there is some loss of thiamin, but otherwise these processes have little adverse effect on the nutrients. Some fish, that are cured and smoked or canned in brine, can contain high levels of sodium (salt). Modern methods of freezing do not affect the nutritive value, and poaching and steaming incur only small losses of vitamins. Between 10 and 30 per cent losses of B-vitamins occur on baking, frying or grilling. For estimating the cooked weight of fish, a loss of about 15 per cent may be assumed on gentle cooking unless frying is used: fish fried in batter and fish products which are fried will gain fat on cooking.

Eggs

IMPORTANCE IN THE DIET

The consumption of eggs has decreased significantly over the last 20 years. The current average consumption is about 2 eggs per person per week. Eggs therefore can still make a small but useful contribution to the daily intakes of vitamin D, retinol, riboflavin, iodine and protein in the average diet and for the elderly they can be an important source of protein, vitamin B_{12} and vitamin D. It used to be thought that eggs were a good source of iron; however, it is now known that the body does not easily absorb the form in which iron occurs in egg yolk.

The shell colour is related to the breed of hen rather than to nutrient content and in this respect it is therefore unimportant; similarly a deep-yellow yolk does not necessarily indicate a high vitamin A content since the pigment is not beta-carotene.

It has been shown that there is no practical difference in the composition of eggs obtained from battery, deep-litter and free-range hens.

To ensure variety in the diet it is wise not to rely too heavily on eggs as an alternative to meat, for example when providing meals for vegetarians.

EFFECTS OF COOKING

When eggs are boiled or fried the proteins coagulate first in the white, at approximately 60°C (140°F), then in the yolk. This property makes eggs suitable for binding dry ingredients together in cooking, and for thickening sauces and soups; the mixture of eggs and milk sets in baked egg custard. Over-cooking causes the proteins to curdle and contract slightly and a yellow watery fluid to separate out; this may occur when scrambling eggs or boiling sauces to which eggs have been added.

The black discoloration that is sometimes present around the yolk of hard-boiled eggs is iron sulphide. This is formed during cooking from hydrogen sulphide in the egg white and iron in the egg yolk. Cooling the eggs in water immediately after cooking can reduce the blackening.

When egg whites are beaten, the proteins hold air to form a stable foam which coagulates or sets at a very low temperature, as in meringues. Eggs are also used for aeration, for example in sponge cakes, and to promote the emulsification of fat, as in mayonnaise. Some of the heat-sensitive B-vitamins are lost during cooking. For example, the average loss of thiamin which results from boiling, frying, poaching and scrambling is between 5 and 15 per cent; similar losses of niacin also occur and slightly higher losses (15-30 per cent) of these and other B-vitamins take place in baked dishes. During frying, the fat content of eggs may be increased by about 50 per cent.

Eggs should be stored in the fridge. Eggs given to infants, pregnant women or to frail older people should be cooked until both the yolk and white are solid to avoid the risk of food poisoning.

Pulses, nuts and seeds

Pulses (legumes) such as dried peas, beans, chickpeas and lentils, and the range of canned pulse products now available, are rich in protein and are an excellent source of fibre. They also contain non-haem iron (page 44) that may be more easily absorbed by the body if pulses are consumed on the same occasion as a good source of vitamin C (like fruits, vegetables or a glass of fruit juice) or by meat. In general they are used as meat alternatives, especially by vegetarians and vegans. They provide more energy and B-vitamins than many vegetables, but do not contain vitamin C. Because their nutrient content differs from that of most other vegetables it is recommended that, however much is eaten, they should only count once towards the recommended five portions of fruit and vegetables per day (see p. 108).

Soya drink (previously known as soya milk) derived from soya beans is used as an animal milk substitute and is sometimes fortified with calcium and sweetened with fruit juice. Soya flour and other products derived from soya are increasingly used in manufactured foods. They are nutritionally valuable, but extra nutrients are added if they are intended to resemble or replace meat (see p. 21).

Nuts, peanuts (which are actually a type of legume) and derived products, such as peanut butter, are rich in fat, especially monounsaturates, and are consequently a concentrated source of energy. They are an excellent source of protein and fibre and a good source of B-vitamins and vitamin E, but contain no vitamin A or C.

Seeds from sunflowers, pumpkins and sesame, and products such as tahini paste from sesame seeds, have a nutritional value similar to nuts.

Cereals

IMPORTANCE IN THE DIET

Cereal grains are a major component of the human diet throughout the world. In Britain, wheat in the form of bread, flour, biscuits, cakes and pasta, together with other cereals such as rice, oatmeal and breakfast cereals, provides about one-third of the total energy, a quarter of the protein and about half of the carbohydrate, fibre and iron in the average adult diet, although the iron is poorly absorbed. Cereals also make a substantial contribution to the intake of many other nutrients, particularly calcium, niacin and thiamin, which are added to most wheat flours, sodium from added salt, and fibre. In general, the common cereals (wheat, oats, barley, rye, maize and rice) contain 65-80 per cent carbohydrate (starch), 7-13 per cent protein, 1-9 per cent fat, 2-15 per cent fibre and approximately 12 per cent moisture in the whole grain. Advances in plant breeding have led to the development of cereal varieties that are richer in lysine; some increases in protein levels may be obtained experimentally by the appropriate use of manures and fertilisers.

Cereals and their products such as bread, pasta and noodles, together with tubers and roots such as yams and potatoes, are starchy foods that should make up about one third of the diet (see the Eatwell plate p. 163)

NUTRIENT LOSSES IN MILLING AND THE COMPOSITION OF WHEAT FLOUR

The distribution of nutrients within the wheat grain is not uniform. The concentration of protein, minerals and vitamins is higher in the germ and outer layers of the grain than in the inner starchy endosperm; thus when wheat is milled to produce white flour a proportion of the nutrients and fibre is discarded with the bran and germ. Owing to the continuing, if decreasing, preference for white flour in the British diet, those nutrients lost in the refining process which are of importance in relation to the diet as a whole are replaced. Similar losses of minerals and vitamins occur in the milling of rice unless it is parboiled, a process which causes nutrients to migrate from the outer to the inner parts of the grain.

The composition of flour in the UK is controlled by Government Regulations (Appendix 8, p. 167-168) which require that all flours contain minimum quantities of two B-vitamins (thiamin and niacin) and iron, corresponding to the levels occurring naturally in 80 per cent extraction flour[1]. These quantities are listed below.

	Per 100g
Iron	1.65 mg
Thiamin (vitamin B_1)	0.24 mg
Niacin	1.60 mg

All wheat flours, with the exception of wholemeal wheat flour, wheat malt flour and self raising flour which has a calcium content of not less than 0.2%, have to be fortified with these nutrients to bring their concentrations to the prescribed levels; wholemeal flours contain more than the specified minimum quantities. In addition calcium carbonate must be added to all flours except wholemeal, wheat meal and certain self-raising flours at the rate of 235 - 390 mg per 100 g.

WHOLEMEAL, BROWN AND WHITE WHEAT FLOURS

The composition of each of these flours varies, but in general wholemeal flour contains somewhat greater amounts of most minerals and several vitamins, particularly of the B group, but less calcium than the flours to which calcium has been added. Wholemeal flour also contains more fibre and phytic acid than brown or white flour. However, apart from the fibre content, nutritional differences between wholemeal and the fortified brown and white flours are unlikely to be of practical significance in a mixed diet.

Traditionally, flours which will produce a large loaf of good quality need to contain sufficient gluten (the protein which is responsible for the bread 'structure' (see also p. 23), either from 'strong' varieties of wheat or else added separately. 'Weak' wheats, such as those grown in the UK, give flours which are more suitable for making biscuits and cakes (but see Chorleywood Bread Process (overleaf).

EFFECTS OF COOKING AND PROCESSING

Cooking causes the starch granules of which cereal carbohydrate is composed to swell and gelatinise, thus making the starch digestible; it also results in a tripling (approximately) of the weight of rice and pasta on boiling as they take up water.

---

[1] The weight of flour obtained from a given weight of cleaned grain, expressed as a percentage, is known as the extraction rate.

Thiamin is the vitamin mainly affected during the baking or processing of cereal products because it is sensitive to heat and destroyed by alkali. The amount lost therefore varies with the cooking time and the final temperature of the cooked food, and whether or not baking powder is used, as for example in soda bread or scones. Riboflavin and niacin are more stable to heat and the loss on baking is small. Of the other unstable vitamins, folate is low in wheat, and vitamin C is only present if added as a flour improver before making bread. It is then destroyed on baking.

In bread-making the yeast gradually ferments the sugars that are formed from the starch in the dough, breaking them down to alcohol and then to carbon dioxide and water, much of which is driven off. The carbon dioxide causes the bread to rise. When water is added to the flour in the preparation of the dough the proteins gliadin and glutenin combine to form gluten. During baking, the yeast is killed and fermentation ceases. The gluten holds the pockets of gas and then coagulates as cooking proceeds, holding the bread in shape. The gelatinised starch in the bread also contributes to loaf structure. The average loss of thiamin in baking bread is about 15 per cent.

About 80 per cent of the bread sold in the UK is made by the *Chorleywood Bread Process* in which addition of certain substances (improvers) to the mix, and the replacement of conventional fermentation of the dough by a few minutes of intense mechanical agitation in special high speed mixers, decreases production time and allows UK and European wheats to be used. The process itself does not affect the nutritional value of bread significantly. However, UK and European wheat flours have lower levels of selenium than are found in the Canadian wheat flour used in conventional methods. This has resulted in decreased average selenium intakes by the UK population, but the significance of this has yet to be determined.

Toast
When bread is toasted the thiamin content is further reduced; the total loss on toasting is about 15 per cent. The heat drives off water from the bread, so that the content of energy and most other nutrients per unit weight increases or remains the same.

Cakes and biscuits
When making a cake, such as a Victoria sponge cake, air is introduced into the mixture by creaming together the fat and sugar. The eggs are lightly beaten to incorporate air before being added to the creamed mixture and the flour is folded in lightly so that this air is not forced out. During cooking the starch gelatinises and the flour and egg proteins coagulate. The loss of thiamin when making cakes and biscuits varies between 20 and 30 per cent.

The relative proportions of fat and sugar to flour and other ingredients are important in giving different cakes and biscuits their characteristic textures and tastes.

Breakfast cereals
The heat treatment used in the preparation of breakfast cereals destroys a large proportion of the thiamin present in the whole grain. In puffed and flaked products it is usually a total loss but the process used in the preparation of

shredded wheat is less drastic and only about half the thiamin is destroyed. Many breakfast cereals are therefore enriched with thiamin, as well as a wide range of other vitamins including folic acid and vitamin B_{12}, and with iron and these products are important sources of nutrients for many people. Sugar, salt and bran are also added to many products; muesli and some other cereal products also have a variety of dried fruits and nuts added. These, and bran-enriched products, provide an excellent source of fibre. Some types of processing lead to an increase in the proportion of starch that is resistant to digestion (see p. 7) and which may have some functions similar to fibre. When porridge is made from coarse oatmeal the cooking loss of thiamin is about 10 per cent.

Roots, tubers and plantains

POTATOES

Importance in the diet

In many diets potatoes provide the main source of vitamin C, even though the vitamin content per unit weight is comparatively low. The amount is highest in new potatoes and falls gradually during post-harvest storage. Instant potato powder and potato flakes or granules are nutritionally equivalent alternatives to fresh potatoes only if the vitamin C and thiamin which are lost in processing are added back to the products. Because of the comparatively large amounts which are eaten, potatoes contribute more protein and iron than do vegetables in the average diet and they are also useful sources of thiamin, niacin and several other nutrients including fibre. Potatoes, other roots and tubers and cereals, are starchy foods that should make up about one third of the diet. Since they have a different role to vegetables in the average diet - that of a staple food - they do not count towards the recommended five portions of fruit and vegetables per day.

Effects of cooking

The digestibility of raw potato starch is very poor, but is greatly improved by cooking. Careless peeling of potatoes that removes a significant proportion of the flesh along with the skin can result in the loss of vitamin C and some minerals. Water-soluble vitamins and some minerals are lost more readily from peeled potatoes than from potatoes cooked in their skins. Average losses of vitamin C from potatoes are:

Method of cooking potatoes	Vitamin C lost (%)
Boiled after peeling	20-50
Boiled in their skins	20-40
Baked in their skins	10-40
Roasted	15-50
Chipped or fried	15-30

If cooked potatoes are mashed and then kept hot, the loss of vitamin C is greater than if they are left whole under similar conditions.

Potato whiteners or sulphite dips prevent the discoloration of raw prepeeled potatoes when they are prepared centrally for distribution to restaurants and other catering establishments, but the amount of thiamin which is lost when the treated potatoes are boiled or fried as chips and subsequently kept hot is greatly increased by this treatment.

The fat content of chips varies from less than 5 per cent of their weight in oven chips to more than 20 per cent in fine-cut French fries. In home prepared or retail chips, it is lowest when the chips are cut large to reduce their surface area, and when the frying oil is kept hot. Fat content can also be reduced by draining the chips on absorbent paper before serving. The amount of the different fatty acids they or other fried staples contain depends on the oil or fat in which they have been fried.

TROPICAL ROOTS AND TUBERS

In the UK, cassava and sweetpotatoes (roots) and yams and eddoes (tubers) are at present eaten in quantity mainly in the ethnic communities particularly by those people originating in Asia, Africa and the West Indies. Plantains (green bananas) are not roots, but fruits. However they occupy a similar place in the diet of communities from Africa and the West Indies. Like potatoes, these foods provide moderate amounts of energy, fibre, vitamins and minerals. Cassava and sweetpotato are similar to potatoes in their vitamin C content, and orange-fleshed, but not white-fleshed, sweetpotatoes can contain substantial quantities of beta-carotene. Due to their nutrient composition and the current limited quantities in which most people in the UK eat them, orange-fleshed sweetpotatoes are classed as a vegetable rather than a staple.

Fruit and vegetables

Importance in the diet

It is recommended that people eat at least five portions of a wide variety of fruits and vegetables each day. This advice is based on many different studies. These have shown consistently that populations that have a high intake of fruit and vegetables have a lower incidence of heart disease, some cancers and other health problems.

However, it appears that it is the mixture of components in fruit and vegetables that is protective rather than any individual component. For this reason it is preferable to eat fruits and vegetables rather than taking dietary supplements.

Portion sizes

All types of fruit and vegetables, fresh, frozen, canned, dried, or pure juices (fruit, vegetable or smoothie) count towards the five or more daily portions. However, since extraction of juice from fruits or vegetables reduces the fibre content and releases non-milk extrinsic sugars (see p. 10) fruit or vegetable juices should not be counted as more than one portion in a day however much is drunk. Smoothies may only count as more than one portion if they contain all of the edible pulped fruit or vegetable.

The following is a guide to portion sizes of fruit and vegetables[2]

ONE portion = 80g = any of these

1 apple, banana, pear, orange or other similar sized fruit
2 plums or similar sized fruit
½ a grapefruit or avocado
1 slice of large fruit, such as melon or pineapple
3 heaped tablespoons of vegetables (raw, cooked, frozen or canned)
A dessert bowl of salad
3 heaped tablespoons of beans and pulses (more than this still counts as a maximum of one portion a day)
3 heaped tablespoons of fruit salad (fresh or canned in fruit juice) or stewed fruit
1 heaped tablespoon of dried fruit (such as raisins and apricots)
1 cupful of grapes, cherries or berries
A glass (150ml) of fruit juice (more than this still counts as a maximum of one portion a day)

Puréed fruits and vegetables are among the first foods given to babies when they are weaned, and it is important that children eat a variety of these foods every day. However, children should only be introduced to five portions a day of these foods gradually between the ages of two and five, adjusting portion sizes to be suitable for the child's age and capacity.

Vegetables

Although they contain 80-95 per cent of water, vegetables supply appreciable quantities of nutrients in the average diet. They are also an important source of fibre (p. 7). Many people do not eat nearly enough vegetables, but their range of colours and textures can be exploited to prepare attractive, appetizing and healthy meals. The composition of a selection of different vegetables is given in Appendix 3. Their nutrient content is influenced by a number of factors during growth and after harvesting and different samples of the same vegetable can vary considerably. For example, the amount of vitamin C will vary with variety, maturity and exposure to sunlight, as well as with the method of handling, the temperature during transport and the delay before the 'fresh' produce is eaten.

GREEN AND SALAD VEGETABLES
Green vegetables, and salad items such as green peppers and tomatoes, are of nutritional importance because of their contribution to the daily intake of vitamin C, beta-carotene (which after absorption is converted to vitamin A in the body),

---

[2] Further details of portion sizes can be found on www.5aday.nhs.uk

folate, iron and other minerals, and fibre. They are especially valuable when eaten raw, as they will suffer no cooking losses; there will, however, be considerable losses of vitamin C and folate in wilted vegetables. Pre-washed salads in atmosphere-controlled packaging are increasingly popular.

ROOT VEGETABLES
Over 60 per cent of the average daily intake of vitamin A (in the form of beta-carotene) is provided by vegetables, much of this by carrots. Sweetpotatoes with orange coloured flesh are excellent sources of beta-carotene. Turnips, swedes and parsnips are comparatively good sources of vitamin C, but they contain no beta-carotene.

Effects of cooking
The main purpose of cooking vegetables is to soften the cellular tissue and to gelatinise any starch that may be present so that they can be digested more easily.

Weight changes in preparation and cooking Peeling and trimming may reduce the purchased weight of some vegetables by up to one-third or more (Appendix 3, p. 143); changes in the weight of most raw vegetables during boiling are small and may be ignored when making calculations from food tables.

Nutrient losses After peeling or shredding, vitamin C is rapidly destroyed by oxidation either directly or by the action of an enzyme present in the plant tissues. This loss can be kept to a minimum by preparing vegetables immediately before use, and by plunging them into boiling water (from which any dissolved oxygen will have been driven off) at the start of the cooking process, when the enzyme will be destroyed.
  During cooking, nutrient losses in vegetables (and to a smaller extent in fruit) are mainly caused by the passage of soluble mineral salts and vitamins from the tissues into the cooking water, and by the destruction of some vitamins by heat. Thus, some of the vitamin C and thiamin are inevitably lost when water is used for cooking because they are both heat-sensitive and water-soluble. It is desirable to use small volumes of water for cooking to keep nutrient losses to the minimum. Green vegetables, which have a large surface area, lose on average between 50 and 75 per cent of their vitamin C during cooking. There is a further loss of vitamin C if there is a delay in service and vegetables are kept hot for any length of time. For example, after being kept hot for 30 minutes, cabbage will provide about 60 per cent of its freshly cooked value, and after an hour, only 40 per cent of its original vitamin C. The currently rare practice of adding sodium bicarbonate to the cooking water to maintain a bright green colour in vegetables accelerates losses of vitamin C. Microwaving is a method of cooking vegetables which heats them rapidly using a minimum quantity of water and conserves their texture and colour.
  It is not necessary to use salt when boiling vegetables.

Effects of processing
The general effects of processing on the nutritive value of foods are discussed on p. 91.
  Freezing does not in itself cause losses of vitamins, but during canning there is some destruction of those vitamins that are unstable to heat (see p. 92-93).

When sulphite is added to dehydrated vegetables to preserve vitamin C and prevent deterioration of quality during storage, most of the thiamin is destroyed. In general, this loss is not serious because in a mixed diet thiamin is obtained from many other foods.

Fruit

In the diet fruit and fruit juices are nutritionally most important as a major source of vitamin C. These foods together now provide nearly 40 per cent of all the vitamin C in the British diet. However, the vitamin C content in different fruits varies widely and will always be lower after cooking. Blackcurrants are exceptionally rich, followed by strawberries, kiwis, other soft fruits, oranges, grapefruit and many fruit juices (but not fruit squash unless it is fortified). Many canned fruits, such as pineapples, mandarin oranges and peaches, also supply moderate quantities of vitamin C. Eating apples, bananas, cherries and rhubarb are examples of fruits which contain much less of the vitamin and which do not in this respect compare favourably with green vegetables. Vitamins and minerals may be added to some fruit products such as apple juice and juice drinks. Fruit juice containers usually carry a nutritional panel in the labelling. Most fruits also contain sugars and small amounts of beta-carotene, other vitamins and minerals. The sugars in unprocessed fruit are considered to be intrinsic sugars and have not been shown to cause dental caries. However, extrinsic sugars are released from the fruit cells during processing in products such as fruit juices and smoothies, which can therefore cause dental caries.

Most commercial *fruit juices* are made from concentrated juice and are preserved by a combination of heating during concentration, and pasteurisation when diluted prior to filling the container. There is now also a fairly large production of freshly squeezed juices prepared directly from the fruit, given a mild pasteurisation treatment, and kept chilled before sale. Juice drinks consist of one or more fruit juices, water, sugar and preservatives. Fruit juices and juice drinks retain their vitamin C well during storage, but once the package is opened the vitamin will slowly be lost through oxidation.

Fruit *smoothies* are blends of one or more pureed fruits; they sometimes have vanilla, honey or yogurt added. They are heat treated and stored similarly to freshly squeezed fruit juices.

Dried fruits such as currants, sultanas, raisins, dates and figs provide energy principally in the form of sugar and are good sources of fibre. They do not contain vitamin C. Prunes and dried apricots are also useful sources of beta-carotene. Dried apricots, figs, prunes, raisins and sultanas are good sources of iron. Dried fruit counts towards the recommended five portions of fruit and vegetables a day, but more of the sugars in dried fruit are likely to be extrinsic (p. 10) than in unprocessed fruit, since they will have been at least partly released from the cells by the drying process. Therefore it is sensible not to eat them too frequently during the day as snacks and to preferably eat them at meal times.

Fat spreads and oils

There is now a wide range of margarines, dairy spreads, and reduced- and lower-fat spreads on the market, all of which can be used as butter substitutes. While some margarines consist of a mixture of animal fats and vegetable oils, others contain vegetable oils with a significant proportion of polyunsaturated fatty acids. Almost any edible oil or fat can be used for making fat spreads.

Varying textures can be produced by mixing oils and fats with differing physical properties and by hydrogenation or hardening of oils. During manufacture the mixture of oils and fats is emulsified with a salt solution and other constituents such as emulsifiers, flavouring and colouring. *Margarine* by law contains a minimum of 80 per cent fat and not more than 16 per cent water.

Dairy spreads contain variable amounts (but less than 80 per cent) of milk fat such as butter or cream. The fat of *blended spreads* is only part milk fat. *Reduced- or low fat spreads* generally vary in fat content from about 20 per cent in a very-low-fat spread to about 40 per cent in a low-fat spread and 60 or 70 per cent in a reduced-fat spread. However, spreads with only 5 per cent fat are now available; these contain a proportion of a fat replacer (see below). Some spreads now contain stanol esters (plant sterols), made from a plant extract, which can help to reduce blood LDL cholesterol levels (see p. 17). Plant sterols lower blood cholesterol levels by reducing the absorption of cholesterol from the intestine. It is advisable for pregnant and breastfeeding women and children under 5 years of age not to consume plant sterols since they can interfere with fat-soluble vitamin absorption.

Vitamins A and D must, by law, be added to margarine for retail sale. The values required are 800 - 1000 µg vitamin A (retinol equivalents) and 7.05 – 8.82 µg vitamin D per 100 g. These vitamins are also frequently added to other fat spreads, but this is not obligatory.

Vegetable oils are produced from a variety of plant parts including seeds (e.g. sunflower, rape (canola)), grains (e.g. maize or corn), pulses (e.g. soya beans, peanuts), fruits (e.g. olive, palm) and fruit kernels (e.g. olive, palm, coconut). They are traditionally extracted by crushing or milling, but nowadays these processes may be replaced or followed by solvent extraction. Vegetable oils vary in the composition of their fatty acids. They may be sold as a single type, or as a blend of several oils. Some oils, such as sunflower, are high in polyunsaturated fatty acids, while others, such as olive and rape (canola) seed oils, are high in monounsaturated fatty acids.

FAT REPLACERS

Dietary advice to reduce the consumption of fat has stimulated research into ways of reducing the fat content of foods by developing fat replacers which have some of the sensory characteristics of fats, but a lower energy value. Salutrim®, made from modified triglycerides, has been approved for use in the EU. Others, including protein-based, carbohydrate-based and sucrose polyester replacers, may be approved for food use in the future.

Sugars and preserves

White sugar provides energy and no other nutrient. Honey and some brown sugars include very small quantities of minerals and certain B-vitamins, but nowhere near enough of the latter to assist with the metabolism of the sugars present. Some preserves contain vitamin C, and chocolate contains iron and other nutrients, but the main function of all these foods in the diet is to increase palatability. Table sugar, honey, syrups and the sugar added to preserves are all non-milk extrinsic sugars (see p. 10) that can cause dental caries if eaten frequently, especially between meals.

Alcohol

The alcohol in alcoholic drinks is rapidly absorbed from the digestive tract and utilised as a source of energy, 1 g of alcohol providing 29 kJ or 7 kcal. Carbohydrate may also be present in varying proportions and this provides additional energy. Consumption of spirits, beer and wine continues to rise and it was reported that in 2000-01 British adults on an average daily basis obtained 635 kJ (153 kcal); 732 kJ (175 kcal) in the case of men, and 270 kJ (65 kcal) in the case of women, from alcohol. This represented 6.5 and 3.9 per cent, respectively, of their total energy intake. Table 30 gives the energy constituents of some alcoholic drinks.

Chronic alcoholics may obtain a large proportion of their energy intake from alcohol and eat very little food. Beer contains significant amounts of riboflavin and niacin, but spirits contain no vitamins; inevitably the displacement of food by alcohol leads to a marked reduction in the intake of protein, vitamins and many other nutrients.

Table 30. Energy constituents of some alcoholic drinks.

| | Average values per 100 ml | | | |
	Alcohol (g)	Carbohydrate (g)	Energy (kJ)	(kcal)
Beer, draught, canned and bottled	2.9	2.2	124	30
Lager	4.0	0.0	121	29
Cider, sweet	3.7	4.3	176	42
Sherry, medium	13.3	5.9	482	116
Red wine	9.6	0.2	283	68
White wine, dry	9.1	0.6	275	66
White wine, sweet	10.2	5.9	394	94
Spirits	31.7	0.0	919	222
Liqueur, low-medium strength	19.8	32.8	1099	262

1 ml of pure alcohol weighs 0.79 g

12 Nutritional value of meals and the whole diet

The balanced diet

No single food contains all the essential nutrients the body needs to be healthy and function efficiently, neither should a single food be considered intrinsically 'healthy' or 'unhealthy', although some foods are more likely to contribute beneficially to a nutritious diet than others. It is the nutritional value of a person's diet as a whole that is important. This depends on the overall mixture or balance of foods that is eaten over a period of time as well as on the needs of the individual eating them. That is why a balanced diet is one that includes a wide variety of foods, so that adequate intakes of all the nutrients are achieved. Scientists have agreed for many years now that some common health problems, including heart disease and stroke, can be diet-related. Too much saturated fat, for example, is recognised as a contributor to heart disease. In this sense a 'balanced' diet also means one with a limited content of fat, which also helps to limit the saturated fat content.

The UK Government has set targets for reductions in the number of people suffering heart disease and stroke and, to help achieve these aims, it will be necessary to reduce fat and particularly saturated fatty acids (p. 12) and salt (p. 82) and to increase the quantity of fruit and vegetables in the average diet of the population. Expert committees regularly review scientific evidence for the relationship between diet and disease. A person's genes influence their risk of developing diet-related diseases, and other lifestyle factors are also regarded as being very important, particularly being physically active and smoking. Diet plays a part in the development or prevention of stroke, since high sodium (salt) intake is associated with a rise in blood pressure (p. 50), which is also influenced by obesity (p. 29) and excessive alcohol intake. Obese people also have an increased risk of heart disease because they are more likely to have raised levels of blood pressure and blood cholesterol. However, sound nutritional practice can help in preventing these problems by developing eating habits that promote the maintenance of good health throughout life. For example, when someone is obese through persistent overeating, only a steady reduction in energy intake or increase in energy expenditure, and not sporadic bouts of starvation or exercise, will lead to weight loss that can be maintained. A vitamin deficiency will not result from a diet that is low or lacking in that vitamin for a few days. Nevertheless, the diet is much more likely to contain enough vitamins, especially vitamin C, if a variety of fruit and vegetables is eaten every day than if these foods are only eaten at infrequent intervals (see also p. 107). It is also now being increasingly recognised that, in addition to vitamins, a large number of other components that occur naturally in fruits and vegetables may contribute towards their protective effect against diet-related diseases. It is recommended that at least five portions of a variety of fruit and vegetables should be eaten each day (see p. 107).

Although heart disease will not result from eating the occasional fat rich meal, it is wise not to consistently include large amounts of fat, especially saturated fatty acids, in the diet. The maintenance of a sensible and regular eating pattern is important for everyone, so that over the long term a person should ensure that their overall diet is balanced in the way described in this manual, particularly someone whose needs are high or whose appetites may be small, such as a young child, a pregnant woman or an elderly person (see Chapter 13). Apart from these vulnerable groups most people can get all the nutrients they need from a balanced diet and do not need dietary supplements. Food is more likely to be enjoyed, rather than treated simply as something to fill up on in a hurry, if people ensure that their diet is made up of a wide range of different foods so that it is varied and interesting.

Meals and choice of foods

A meal can be arbitrarily defined as the amount of food eaten at one period of time and which provides 850 kJ (200 kcal) or more. This definition covers much more than the popular meaning of the word, which is that of hot, cooked food eaten while sitting down. Different people may eat quite different numbers of meals per day, the arrangements being determined by custom, lifestyle and by working conditions. Many people now do not follow the traditional pattern of three main meals and one or more snacks, but 'graze' or 'snack' at frequent intervals throughout the day. There is evidence that the number of meals taken in a day (and consequently the amount of food eaten at one time) influences the pattern of utilisation of nutrients by the body. However, the balance of nutrients achieved over a period of time is undoubtedly more important in determining a person's nutritional status than the frequency of eating occasions. Nevertheless, it is sensible to try and eat one or more balanced meals each day. Although the amounts of nutrients in different meals may vary, the total intake of each nutrient should meet an individual's needs, ideally each day but certainly over a period of a week, if the food eaten is to be fully satisfactory for health.

Apart from breast milk, which satisfies all a baby's needs for the first six months of life, no single food provides all the nutrients we require. The easiest way of providing an adequate mixture and balance of all the nutrients is to eat a wide variety of foods chosen from among four main groups: starchy foods, vegetables and fruit, dairy products and meat or meat alternatives.

People who eat sweets, cakes, biscuits or chocolate between meals or as constant snacks will probably have a reduced appetite for cereals, vegetables or meat at the next meal with the result that they may have a low intake of some nutrients. They may also be more prone to dental decay, which can develop from frequent eating of sweet foods. Eating large quantities of high energy foods at or between meals can result in an undesirable increase in weight if the total daily energy intake exceeds the energy used up and, if these foods are high in saturated fatty acids, may lead to raised blood cholesterol levels and eventually to the development of heart disease. For adults, the heavy consumption of alcoholic drinks can result in excess energy intake.

BREAKFAST

Because of the length of time since the previous meal, and the consequent low blood sugar level in the morning, it is desirable to eat breakfast every morning. It is particularly important for children, and people in demanding jobs, to have a good breakfast as this helps to keep them alert during the morning. Young children may not be able to satisfy their needs during the rest of the day if breakfast is missed; others may be tempted to fill up on nutrient-poor foods on the way to school or during the morning. Two possible light breakfasts, both commonly eaten in Britain, are shown in Table 31. Breakfast 2 provides less fat and saturated fatty acids and much more fibre and vitamin C than Breakfast 1. Both provide adequate amounts of energy, protein and a wide variety of vitamins and minerals (not shown). Breakfast 2 also provides two of the five recommended portions of fruit and vegetables for the day (a banana and a glass of orange juice). Substituting a cereal with little or no sodium (salt), like shredded wheat or some types of muesli, for those shown in Table 31, can reduce the sodium content of these breakfasts. A person who feels unable to eat breakfast immediately on getting up should be encouraged to take a nutritious snack as soon as possible during the morning. Breakfast clubs in schools can alleviate the hunger felt by children who do not eat breakfast at home and, if healthy choices are provided, can help improve the nutritional quality of their overall daily diet.

Calculation of nutrients in prepared dishes and meals, using food tables

DISHES

Appendix 3 gives the nutrient composition of many of the ingredients that may be used in mixed dishes. From the recipe, the approximate nutritional value of a dish can then be worked out by arithmetic. To illustrate this, the calculation of the nutritional value of a home-made Quiche Lorraine is shown in Table 32. An allowance has been made for the change in weight and probable loss of folate and vitamin C during cooking.

MEALS

It is not uncommon to have a choice between two types of meal: for example, one could be a cooked meal and the other a sandwich-based meal. Many people may now eat the latter at midday rather than the former. Some may not consider that they had eaten a meal at all if a sandwich meal is chosen. Table 33 compares the nutrient content of ham sandwiches, a low-fat fruit yogurt and a small glass of orange juice with that of roast chicken, oven chips, peas, canned pineapple and coffee with reduced fat milk (as calculated from the figures given in Appendix 3). It can be seen that the two meals have a very similar energy value, and similar saturated fatty acid, vitamin A and folate contents. This particular snack meal has a lower iron content than the cooked meal, but is richer in calcium and vitamin C. It contains less fibre and will contain considerably more sodium unless the cooked meal is salted during cooking or at the table.

A cold or packed meal is thus not necessarily inferior to a cooked meal; the nutritional values of both depend on the quantity and nutrient content of the items within them. A hot, cooked meal can, however, be comforting on a cold day.

Allowance for waste

The calculation of the nutritional value of a meal or a diet as actually eaten cannot be made directly from the total amounts of the foods bought from the shops, nor from the total food used in the kitchen. There is always a proportion of waste for which allowance must be made, that is:

1. *Inedible waste*, e.g. egg shells, potato peelings, outer leaves of cabbages, orange peel, bacon rinds, bones and gristle of meat, etc. (See Table 34).
2. *Edible waste*

(a) *Preparation losses*, e.g. batter left in mixing bowls, fat trimmed from meat or left in frying pans, crusts from bread, spilt milk.
(b) *Table waste*, e.g. scraps left on plates.
(c) *Pet food*, e.g. edible scraps fed to domestic pets, garden birds, ducks.
(d) Edible food which has 'gone bad' and is discarded.

INEDIBLE WASTE

Average figures for the inedible waste associated with different foods are given in Appendix 3 as a percentage of the product as listed. For example, 34 per cent of bananas (item 162), as purchased, consist of skin that is not eaten.

The food tables throughout this manual always give the nutrients per 100 g of 'edible portion', and if they are used for calculating the nutritional value of foods where only the purchased weight is known, the percentage of inedible waste must be deducted. For example, to calculate the energy value of a 1 kg (purchased weight) of bananas:

Edible weight = $(100 - 34)$ x 10 = 660 g

Energy value $= \dfrac{660}{100}$ x (kJ per 100 g from Appendix 3)

$\qquad\qquad = \dfrac{660}{100}$ x 403 = 2660 kJ (a similar calculation can be carried out using carried out using kcal per 100 g from Appendix 3)

Table 31. Comparison of two breakfasts

	Weight (g)	Energy (kJ)	Energy (kcal)	Total Sugars (g)	Protein (g)	Fat (g)	Saturated fatty acids (g)	Fibre (g)	Sodium (mg)	Vitamin C (mg)
Light breakfast 1										
Cornflakes	30	480	113	2.5	2.4	0.3	0.1	0.3	300	0
Sugar	10	168	39	10.5	0.0	0.0	0.0	0.0	1	0
Milk, whole	100	274	66	4.5	3.3	3.9	2.5	0.0	43	2
White bread (large loaf, 1 medium slice), toasted	27	307	72	1.1	2.6	0.5	0.1	0.6	152	0
Fat spread (60% fat), polyunsaturated	9	205	50	0.1	0.0	5.5	1.0	0.0	64	0
Marmalade	15	167	39	10.4	0.0	0.0	0.0	0.0	10	2
Milk (whole) in 2 cups of tea	50	137	33	2.3	1.7	2.0	1.3	0.0	21	1
Total		1738	412	31.4	10.0	12.2	5.0	0.9	591	5
Light breakfast 2										
Wheat biscuits, 2	40	599	141	2.0	4.5	1.1	0.2	3.9	108	0
Milk, semi-skimmed	100	195	46	4.7	3.4	1.7	1.1	0.0	43	1
Banana, small	80	322	76	16.7	1.0	0.2	0.1	0.9	1	9
Wholemeal bread (large loaf, 1 thick slice), toasted	40	434	102	1.3	4.5	1.2	0.2	2.4	228	0
Low fat spread (35-40% fat),	9	135	33	0.1	0.4	3.4	0.8	0.0	59	0
Marmalade	15	167	39	10.4	0.0	0.0	0.0	0.0	10	2
Milk (semi-skimmed) in 2 cups of tea	60	117	28	2.8	2.0	1.0	0.7	0.0	26	1
Orange juice, average glass	150	229	54	13.2	0.8	0.2	0.0	0.2	15	59
Total		2198	519	51.2	16.6	8.8	3.1	7.4	490	72

Manual of Nutrition

Table 32. Nutrients in a home-made Quiche Lorraine

	Weight (g)	Energy (kJ)	Energy (kcal)	Protein (g)	Fat (g)	Saturated fatty acids (g)	Carbohydra (g)
Flour mixture:							
White	67	972	229	6.3	0.9	0.1	52.1
Wholemeal	67	883	208	8.5	1.5	0.2	42.8
Margarine, polyunsaturated	66	2024	492	0.0	54.6	11.2	0.1
Eggs	100	627	151	12.5	11.2	3.2	0.0
Milk, semi-skimmed	207	404	95	7.0	3.5	2.3	9.7
Streaky Bacon	100	1142	276	15.8	23.6	8.2	0.0
Cheddar cheese	100	1725	416	25.4	34.9	21.7	0.1
Whole quiche, cooked	527	7777	1867	75.5	130.2	46.9	104.8
Per 100g		1476	354	14.3	24.7	8.9	19.9

The quiche weight (527 g) is less than the sum of the ingredients (707 g) owing to the loss of moisture on cooking.
50% of folate deducted to allow for loss on cooking; 50% of vitamin C deducted to allow for loss on cooking.

Table 33. Comparison of the nutritional value of a snack and a cooked meal

	Weight (g)	Energy (kJ)	Energy (kcal)	Protein (g)	Fat (g)	Saturate fatty ac (g)
Snack meal						
Bread, wholemeal (2 slices)	72	664	156	6.8	1.8	0.4
Fat spread, blended, 70-80% fat, polyunsaturated	14	391	95	0.1	10.5	3.6
Ham, sliced (2 slices)	46	207	49	8.5	1.5	0.5
Pickle, sweet	20	121	28	0.1	0.0	0.0
Yogurt, low fat, fruit	125	414	97	5.3	1.4	1.0
Orange juice	150	230	54	0.8	0.1	0.0
Total		2027	479	21.6	15.3	5.5
Cooked meal						
Roast chicken, meat only	100	742	177	27.3	7.5	2.9
Chips, oven baked	165	1134	267	5.3	6.9	3.0
Peas, frozen, boiled in unsalted water	80	233	55	4.8	0.7	0.2
Pineapple, canned in juice	80	160	38	0.2	0.0	0.0
Coffee, infusion, cup	190	15	4	0.4	0.0	0.0
Milk, semi-skimmed	30	59	14	1.0	0.5	0.3
Total		2343	555	39.0	15.6	6.4

118

ibre g)	Calcium (mg)	Iron (mg)	Sodium (mg)	VIitamin A (retinol equivalent) (µg)	Folate (µg)	Riboflavin (mg)	Niacin equivalent (mg)	Vitamin C (mg)
2.1	94	1.3	2	0	15	0.02	2.4	0.0
5.0	25	2.6	2	0	38	0.06	5.5	0.0
0.0	3	0.2	449	484	0	0.00	0.0	0.0
0.0	57	1.9	140	190	50	0.47	3.8	0.0
0.0	248	0.0	89	42	12	0.50	1.9	2.0
0.0	6	0.5	1260	0	3	0.14	7.4	0.0
0.0	739	0.3	723	388	31	0.39	6.9	0.0
3.1	1172	6.8	2665	1104	75	1.58	27.9	1.0
1.5	222	1.3	506	209	14	0.30	5.3	0.2

Carbohydrate (g)	Fibre (g)	Calcium (mg)	Iron (mg)	Sodium (mg)	Vitamin A (retinol equivalent) (µg)	Folate (µg)	Vitamin C (mg)
30.2	3.6	76	1.7	351	0	29	0.0
0.2	0.0	2	0.0	94	89	0	0.0
0.5	0.0	3	0.3	552	0	9	0.0
7.2	0.2	3	0.1	322	8	0	0.0
17.1	0.3	175	0.1	78	13	20	1.0
13.2	0.2	15	0.3	15	4	27	59.0
68.4	4.3	274	2.5	1412	114	85	60.0
0.0	0.0	17	0.8	100	24	10	0.0
49.2	3.3	20	1.3	87	0	35	20.0
7.8	4.1	28	1.3	2	76	26	10.0
9.8	0.4	6	0.4	1	2	1	9.0
0.6	0.0	6	0.2	0	0	0	0.0
1.4	0.0	36	0.0	13	6	2	0.0
68.8	7.8	113	4.0	203	108	74	39.0

Typical values for the percentage of inedible waste in selected foods are shown in Table 34, but in reality values vary with the exact nature of the food and with its quality. For example, they vary between different cuts and joints of meat and between different sizes and varieties of orange. The values given must therefore be used with discretion.

Table 34. Percentage of inedible waste from food as purchased

Food	%
Chicken, drumsticks, roasted	37
Lamb chop, loin	22
Kipper, grilled	37
Sardines, canned in oil	18
Tuna, canned in brine	19
Eggs, chicken, whole	11
Potatoes, new, with skin	11
Potatoes, old, with skin	20
Beans, red kidney, canned	36
Beetroot, boiled	20
Cabbage	23
Celery	9
Courgettes	12
Lettuce	26
Mushrooms, unpeeled	3
Onions	9
Peppers, green	16
Peas, canned	35
Sweet corn kernels, canned	18
Watercress	38
Apples, eating	11
Avocado	29
Bananas	34
Blackcurrants	2
Cherries	17
Dates, dried, with stones	16
Grapefruit	32
Grapes	5
Kiwi fruit	14
Mangoes	32
Melon, Honeydew	37
Oranges	30
Peaches	10
Pears	9
Plums	6
Strawberries	5
Almonds, with shells	63

Fresh produce unless specified.

EDIBLE WASTE

It is often difficult for practical reasons to measure the weight of food actually eaten, for example by a particular individual in a large family or when a meal is eaten away from home. Estimates of portion sizes and of the loss of edible food may then need to be made before the nutritional adequacy of any diet can be worked out. The average wastage of food in the home in cooking, on plates and from food given to pets has been found to be between 5 and 10 per cent, but of course the amount varies from food to food and from family to family. Wastage can also be high in some catering establishments.

Planning balanced meals and nutritionally adequate diets

The provision of palatable and acceptable meals must be the first consideration; only if foods are eaten, and not wasted, can planning for good nutrition be effective.

A balanced meal is one which provides adequate amounts of protein and of all the minerals and vitamins as well as energy. It should also provide fibre, and should be limited in its fat, sugar and salt content. At least one balanced meal should be eaten every day.

The main sources of each nutrient are discussed in Chapters 2, 3, 4, 7 and 8, and the detailed composition of a range of foods is given in Appendix 3. Most foods contain a wide variety of nutrients, and most minerals and vitamins are present in a wide variety of commonly available foods. Thus the simplest way to meet nutritional standards is to eat a varied diet containing a wide selection of different types of food.

Experience and custom have influenced food choice in such a way that traditional meals are generally nutritionally satisfactory as well as good to eat; nevertheless to be sure that this is maintained, now that we rely to a greater extent on snacks and convenience foods, certain rules can be followed. To help make this easier, the Government has produced a set of 8 tips for eating well and a pictorial guide to a healthy diet called the Eatwell plate (see Appendix 6). In general:

(a) Starchy foods, such as bread, rice, potatoes and pasta which provide energy, fibre, vitamins and minerals, should form the main part of most meals and snacks, making up about one third of the total food intake.

(b) The daily diet should contain at least five portions of a variety of fruit and vegetables, which are good sources of some vitamins and minerals not commonly found in other foods, and of fibre. These should also make up about one third of the dietary intake.

(c) Moderate amounts of foods selected from meat (trimmed of fat), fish, eggs, pulses, nuts, and moderate amounts of reduced fat versions of milk and dairy products, all rich in protein, vitamins and minerals should accompany the starchy foods and fruit and vegetables in a meal.

(d) Foods rich in energy, such as butter, margarine, reduced-fat spreads, cream, fried foods, jam, cakes, pastries, biscuits and other foods rich in fat and sugars, and alcoholic drinks, should be consumed infrequently or only in limited amounts which will satisfy appetite and maintain correct body weight. It is satisfactory if this balance is achieved over the course of a week or so.

The Reference Nutrient Intakes of selected major nutrients for groups of people of different ages are given on p. 78, and these figures may be used as a guide when planning diets. The Dietary Reference values for fat and carbohydrate for adults are summarised in Table 26 on p. 79. As a rule of thumb, on average, fat should not provide more than 35 per cent of dietary energy for adults, nor saturated fatty acids more than 10 per cent of dietary energy. By implication, the total carbohydrate in the diet should provide about 50 per cent of the food energy, with no more than about 10 per cent coming from non-milk extrinsic sugars. Children under five years of age who are not able to eat large quantities of bulky foods, may not obtain sufficient energy unless they are given energy-dense foods. It is therefore not wise to limit their fat intake too much (note that human breast milk derives 54 per cent of its energy from fat and 26 per cent from saturated fatty acids).

The adult diet should provide 18 g per day of fibre as non-starch polysaccharides. Whole meal versions of cereals provide more fibre than refined products.

The Reference Nutrient Intakes of sodium for adults and children, as shown on p. 78, can be readily achieved from the salt already present in food. Since 75% of salt is already in the food we purchase, people should try to eat fewer salty foods, but also use less salt in cooking and at the table. It is not always easy to tell by taste alone whether a food is high in salt. Checking the nutrition label on a product will be very helpful in choosing a lower sodium food (see also Appendix 6). For example if a 500 g ready-prepared meal contains 0.5 g sodium (1.25 g salt) per 100 g, it would provide 2.5 g sodium (6 g salt). This is the maximum amount adults should be having in a whole day. Other practical ways to help to reduce salt intakes include: using herbs (fresh or dried) and spices to flavour dishes, choosing products that are marked 'reduced salt' or 'no added salt'; cutting down on salty snacks such as crisps, salted nuts and heavily salted foods; choosing lower salt stock cubes.

In practice it will be found that certain meals such as the traditional Sunday lunch are likely to be rich in fat and other nutrients whereas others, including breakfasts for many people, will provide a counterbalance. It is the total nutrient intake over at least one day (as in the example given on page 138), and preferably a week, that should be assessed. And even then it is the balance of the diet in the longer term which is really important for health.

Planning meals in relation to cost

Within this general framework it is usually necessary to consider the relative cost of different sources of nutrients. Allowance must also be made for the effects of cooking on nutritive value.

Great savings in the cost of eating can be made with a thorough knowledge of food composition and nutritional value for money. For example, cheaper cuts of lean meat have practically the same nutritional value as the more expensive cuts although they may take longer to cook. Many meat products also provide good nutritional value for money. However, fatty meat and some meat products may prove relatively expensive if large quantities of fat have to be trimmed off before cooking or discarded after cooking. Again, cheaper oily fish such as mackerel have a similar nutritional value to a more expensive oily fish such as salmon. Buying vegetables and fruit in season is usually less expensive, and frozen vegetables can be good value as there is no waste associated with preparing them and they often have a higher content of nutrients than fresh vegetables which have been stored at room temperature for some time. Fresh citrus fruits are very convenient sources of vitamin C and are also fairly cheap. Cheese, eggs or pulses can take the place of meat in a main course.

Section 3 of Appendix 4 shows how a comparison can be made between the amounts of protein, vitamins or other nutrients bought for one monetary unit (in this case a penny) for any food by using the food composition tables and the price of the food. The precise relationship between foods will vary according to the time of year and current prices. It is important to realise that a cheap source of one nutrient may not be a cheap food in the context of the whole diet, as with sugar where only one nutrient is supplied. Bread, pasta, rice, breakfast cereals, milk, cheese, offals, oily fish, potatoes, peas and beans, on the other hand, all supply several nutrients cheaply and are thus very good value for money.

Planning meals for the week ahead is really important in food budgeting. Careful shopping, preparation and storage of food, and a knowledge of basic cookery skills all play a part in using the available money to the best advantage.

13 Needs of particular groups of people

Infants and young children

Babies are unique in that they must rely on a single food, milk, to satisfy all their nutritional needs. Breast milk is ideal for several reasons:

(a) All the nutrients are present in the right amount for human infants (children less then 12 months old), and in a readily absorbed form. Those nutrients which are low, such as iron and copper, are those which are already stored in large amounts in the infant's liver.

(b) It contains several natural agents which protect against disease.

(c) It is clean and cannot be prepared incorrectly.

A mother should therefore try to breastfeed her baby, ideally for 6 months. There are benefits from breastfeeding even if the mother only breastfeeds for a few weeks, but the longer breastfeeding can continue the greater the benefits. Few mothers are unable to breastfeed. Those who cannot do so for medical reasons or who prefer not to should use formulas. These are usually based on cow's milk, which has been modified so that the formulas are more like human milk. Since the immature kidneys of young infants are unable to adapt to high concentrations of protein and some minerals it is very important to make up these feeds exactly according to the instructions so that they are not too concentrated. Also formulas should also not be diluted more than stated in the instructions since the formula will then not contain enough energy or nutrients for the baby's needs. Hydrolysed protein infant formulas may be prescribed by a GP if a baby has an allergy to cows' milk. Milks based on goats' milk protein have not been approved for use by the European Food Safety Authority for babies under a year old, and so should not be used for babies. Soya-based infant formulas should only be used on the advice of a GP or health visitor. Babies who are allergic to cows' milk proteins may also be allergic to goats' milk or soya proteins.

When a baby is around six months old solid foods can be introduced in addition to breast or formula milk. Before this, a baby's immature digestive system may be at risk. Solid foods should never be introduced before 4 months of age. There is no advantage to the baby to do so and there may be some risks of becoming obese. Foods that can cause an allergic reaction in some infants and should not be given under 6 months are: wheat-based foods and other foods containing gluten — including bread, wheat flour, breakfast cereals and rusks; nuts and seeds — including peanuts, peanut butter and other nut spreads; eggs; fish and shell fish. Children who face the highest risk of peanut allergy are those with parents, brothers or sisters who have certain allergic conditions, such as asthma, eczema, or hayfever. For this group, breast feeding mothers may wish to avoid eating peanuts or their products and not to give peanuts or, foods containing peanuts (such as peanut butter) or unrefined cold-pressed groundnut (peanut) oil, until the child is at least three years old.

From about 6 months onwards the mother may gradually introduce infant cereal foods, puréed fruit and vegetables, whole egg (cooked until solid), and even finely blended or minced meat (using no added salt or sugar). By about 12 - 18 months, the infant can eat a mixed diet not very different from that of the rest of the family. Foods high in salt such as cheese, bacon or sausages, or processed foods, such as pasta sauces or breakfast cereals, that are not made specifically for babies are best avoided for infants who should have less than 1 g of salt a day before 6 months and no more than 1 g per day at 7 – 12 months.

Whole, pasteurised cow's, goat's or sheep's milk do not contain the right balance of nutrients for infants and are particularly low in iron, but can be given as a main drink after the age of one year. Above the age of 2, semi-skimmed milk may be introduced as long as a child is eating well. Skimmed milk is not suitable for children under 5. Once the diet has become more varied, infants can be given extra drinks of cooled, boiled water in hot weather, but sugary drinks and juices can harm developing teeth.

Studies have shown that a significant proportion of infants and young children between 9 months and 3½ years of age have low iron intakes (below the Lower Reference Nutrient Intake, see p. 77). Although it has not yet been established whether children with habitually low intakes are deficient in iron, it is wise to include rich sources of iron among the foods provided for this age group. Some good sources of iron are listed in Table 10 (p. 45).

Children under 5, because of their smaller size compared with adults, and correspondingly smaller stomachs, should not be given high-fibre foods such as high fibre breakfast cereals, wholemeal bread or pasta and brown rice. It makes it hard for them to consume enough energy and can reduce the amounts of minerals they absorb.

Vitamin drops should be given to children until they are 5 years old, unless they are really good eaters on a varied diet. Drops containing vitamins A, C and D are provided free under Healthy Start[1] for children aged 6 months to 4 years in those families claiming certain benefits. Fluoride supplements (available as licensed medicines) may be useful in areas where the drinking water is low in fluoride.

School children

School children are growing fast and are also very active. Tables 24 and 25 give the Estimated Average Requirements (EAR) for energy, and Reference Nutrient Intakes (RNI) for major nutrients for groups of children of different ages, and show that these are high in relation to their body size compared with those of adults. For example, the EAR for 7 - to 10 - year-old girls for energy and their RNI for thiamin are nearly as high as those for grown women in most occupations. The big appetites of some children usually

---

[1] Healthy Start replaced the Welfare Food Scheme in 2006. It covers the whole of the UK.

reflect a real nutritional need rather than greed. Because of their smaller size compared with adults, and correspondingly smaller stomachs, it is important that children should eat meals that are not too bulky. Bread, milk, cheese, meat, fish, liver, eggs, fruit, green vegetables and potatoes are all excellent sources of a number of nutrients. Milk, whether whole, semi-skimmed or skimmed, is one of the best sources of calcium, riboflavin and protein.

The incidence of overweight and obesity in children has increased significantly in recent years (see p. 29). Therefore it is important that children are taught sensible eating habits from an early age, both at home and at school: biscuits, sweets, soft drinks, chips and crisps should not displace other more useful foods too often. In the school setting, children should be able to perceive that a healthy eating message is conveyed right across the school, not only through the taught curriculum, but also in the food provided in the school canteen, breakfast clubs, tuck shops and vending machines.

Children's dental health has significantly improved since the 1970s due to the increasing use of fluoride toothpaste. However, sweet and sticky foods, snacks and sugary soft drinks, consumed frequently between meals, are one cause of the dental decay still found in many British school children. Children should be encouraged to clean their teeth twice every day with a fluoride toothpaste.

It is important that children are discouraged from acquiring a taste for salty foods since those aged between 4 - 6 years should have no more than 3 g per day, 7 - 10 years olds no more than 5 g per day and that children of 11 years and over should be consuming no more than 6 g per day (see also p. 50). At present children on average may be consuming significantly more than these targets.

Adolescents

The nutrient needs of adolescents are higher in many respects than those of any other group. Healthy adolescents have large appetites and it is important that they should satisfy them with food of high nutritional value in the form of well-balanced meals rather than by too many snacks rich in fat, sugar or salt. Overweight and obesity among school children is common and increasing and may continue into adult life. It is more sensible to prevent obesity than try to correct it by periodically eating little or no food; excessive dieting can be dangerous. There is also evidence that adolescent obesity is partly due to a general decrease in physical activity and hence in energy expenditure rather than to an excessive energy intake. Knowledge of nutrition and the incentive to apply this knowledge in practice is likely to benefit the health of young people for the rest of their lives.

Adolescents are known to have low intakes of several micronutrients. They also are reported to have low plasma vitamin D. Many adolescents, particularly teenage girls have low intakes of calcium, magnesium and zinc and iron combined with poor vitamin D status.

The late stage of adolescence is an important time for increasing bone density and a lack of calcium, magnesium and vitamin D at this crucial time may result in an increase in fracture later in life. It may be advisable for pregnant adolescents to have calcium intakes higher than the Reference Nutrient Intake (p. 78), although an increment above the RNI is not necessary for other pregnant women (see overleaf). Poor intakes of micronutrients during adolescence and early adulthood can result in low stores of nutrients that can later result in young women being more at risk of giving birth to a low birth weight baby. Adolescent girls who become pregnant are at particular risk of developing nutrient deficiencies, needing additional nutrients for their baby's growth as well as for their own. Infants of adolescent mothers are more likely to be born small and are more at risk of several disabilities[2]. It is particularly important that all teenage girls of childbearing age eat folate-rich foods, such as broccoli, oranges, yeast extract and fortified foods like breakfast cereals and some breads. They should also take a daily supplement of 0.4 mg folic acid, since there may be a risk of an unplanned pregnancy and the possibility of a baby being born with a neural tube defect (see p. 67).

Adults

Many adults in Britain are more likely to be at risk of over nutrition than of under nutrition (see p. 29). Those adults who wish to reduce their intakes of energy to help maintain a healthy weight or to reduce their intakes of saturated fatty acids or salt to reduce their risk of premature heart disease will find information throughout this manual which will help them to achieve this. Anyone needing to make changes to their diet will find these easier to follow if they are shared with, or supported by, other members of the family or friends. There is also information for those who wish to reduce their intakes of sugars and to increase their intake of fibre.

In general, healthy, well-balanced diets are high in starchy foods and fruit and vegetables, contain moderate amounts of meat or its alternatives and milk and dairy foods and only small quantities of foods with high concentrations of fat (especially saturated fat), salt and sugar. The carbohydrate from cereal products including bread, rice and pasta, and from potatoes or other tubers such as yams, is needed to make good the energy lost from any reduction in fats and sugars. These foods also contribute fibre to the diet and are important sources of several nutrients. It is also recommended that people eat at least two portions of fish a week, one of which should be oily fish. Fish is an excellent source of protein and it contains essential vitamins, and minerals such as selenium and iodine. White fish such as cod, haddock and plaice are very low in fat. Oily fish, however, is rich in beneficial omega-3 fatty acids and is a good source of vitamins A and D.

It is always wise to evaluate the whole diet before making any changes so that the intake of other nutrients, as well as the nutrient of concern, and the foods that chiefly contribute to these intakes, are known. There would be little point, for example, in reducing an individual's fat intake further if their diet is already low in fat, or of reducing their intake of a favourite food if this contributes little to their overall fat intake. It is recommended that reducing fat intakes should not result in

---

[2] Under Healthy Start, all girls under 18 who become pregnant are entitled to free vitamin supplements and vouchers to purchase milk, fruit and vegetables, as well as infant formula milk when the baby is born.

higher intakes of foods rich in sugars or salt. Adults should aim to eat no more than 6g of salt each day. The majority of salt is found in manufactured foods and care should be taken when purchasing prepared foods in addition to taking care with the salt added at the table or in cooking.

It is also important to keep alcohol consumption under control, since the energy contained in alcohol can contribute significantly to overall energy intake. Regular consumption of between 3 and 4 units a day or less for men and 2 and 3 units a day or less for women will not significantly increase the risk to a person's health over time. Drinking more than this on a regular basis over time, however, brings increasing risks to health. It is best for women who are pregnant or trying to get pregnant to stop drinking alcohol all together, for those who do drink, they should have no more than 1 or 2 units of alcohol once or twice a week. Light drinking of between 1 and 2 units a day, however, can exert a beneficial protective effect against coronary heart disease for people at risk, namely men over forty and women who have gone through the menopause. A unit of alcohol is half a pint of beer, a small glass of sherry, a glass of wine or a single measure of spirits.

Pregnancy and lactation

A woman's nutritional needs increase during pregnancy and lactation (p. 77 and 78). This is not only because her diet must provide for the growth and development of her child, but also because other physiological changes occur to ensure that sufficient nutrients are available for the child (such as the laying down of new tissues in the woman's own body) and that the mother has enough energy to carry the extra weight. Much of the weight gain during the early part of pregnancy is due to the accumulation of fat, which provides an energy store to meet the additional demands of the growing foetus and the breastfed infant.

Approximate weight of a foetus and infant at various ages

Conception	0 kg
4½ months pregnancy	0.5 kg
9 months pregnancy (birth)	3.5 kg
4½ months after birth	7 kg

It is most important that the mother's diet contains sufficient energy, protein, iron, calcium, folate and vitamins C and D (and liquid during lactation) for building the baby's muscular tissues, bones and teeth, and for the formation of haemoglobin; if it does not, her own stores of nutrients may be reduced.[3] Some good sources of these nutrients are given in Part 1. In practice most of these extra nutrients will be obtained simply by satisfying the appetite with a good mixed diet including plenty of bread, fruit and vegetables, dairy products and meat or its alternatives. Extra folic acid/folate before and during pregnancy is needed by some women to decrease

---

[3] Pregnant women who qualify for certain benefits are eligible for vouchers to purchase fruit and vegetables, milk and infant formula milk under Healthy Start.

the risk of occurrence of neural tube defects in their babies. As it is not known who is at risk, in the case of first-time pregnancies or those with previous normal pregnancies, all women planning a pregnancy are advised to take a daily supplement of 0.4 mg of folic acid before becoming pregnant as well as eating folate-rich foods. Those who have already had an affected child should take 4 or 5 mg folic acid each day. Pregnant women are also recommended to take a supplement of 10 μg of vitamin D throughout pregnancy and lactation. An additional 550 mg per day of calcium is recommended during lactation, but no increase is needed during pregnancy since the body undergoes various adaptations including increased calcium absorption; (however, see adolescents p. 126). Special supplements of iron may also be recommended during pregnancy and free vitamin supplements are available to those on certain benefits under Healthy Start. However, pregnant women are advised not to take supplements containing vitamin A or eat foods such as liver that may be extremely rich in vitamin A, except on the advice of their doctor, due to the possible risk of birth defects (see p. 58). A good knowledge of nutrition is invaluable during pregnancy and lactation and will also help the mother to teach sound eating habits to her child in due course.

Older people

There is very little difference between the nutritional requirements of most older people and the younger adult. However, as age progresses and body weight and energy expenditure decrease, people tend to eat less and hence may find it difficult to satisfy all the nutrient requirements. It is important, therefore, that older people are encouraged to maintain a good energy intake unless they are obese. They should also have foods that are concentrated sources of protein, vitamins and minerals. The EARs (see p. 77) for energy for populations of people aged 60 or over are shown in Table 24. A healthy weight can be more readily maintained and recovery from illness or injury will be more rapid if older people are also encouraged to take plenty of gentle exercise. It has been recommended that older people should adopt diets that will help to moderate their blood cholesterol levels to reduce their risk of heart disease. As with younger adults, therefore, older people should not eat too much saturated fat, should aim to eat meals based on starchy foods and try to eat at least 5 portions a day of a variety of fruit and vegetables. Encouraging them to include oily fish in their diets would help to reduce their risk of thrombosis (development of a blood clot which may block narrowed arteries and result in a heart attack). It has also been recommended that, on average, older people should follow the DRV for non-milk extrinsic sugars which would help them to retain their own teeth (for those without dentures or with only partial dentures), consume a more varied diet than would be possible with high sugar intakes, and prevent possible disorders of their metabolism arising from a high sucrose load. However, when very elderly people are unwell, sugar in amounts additional to recommendations may help to make their food more palatable and encourage them to eat. Foods rich in fibre can also help to prevent constipation.

Those who live alone should be encouraged to prepare at least one meal a day of good nutritional quality, stressing that this does not necessarily have to be a hot meal, and to supplement this with foods such as milk, cheese, yogurt, eggs, breakfast cereals, bread, and fruits or fruit juices rich in vitamin C which need little preparation. It is a good idea, for those times when an elderly person is unwell or when the weather is bad and they are unable to shop, to have a store cupboard of essential items such as powdered or UHT milk, breakfast cereals, cans of fish such as sardines, canned fruit, vegetables, pulses and milk puddings, UHT fruit juices and dried fruit. Items such as frozen ready meals and a supply of bread and vegetables can be kept where a freezer is available.

Older people are at greater risk of osteoporosis, therefore it is important that they should ensure that they get sufficient vitamin D. Whenever possible, older people should go outside for a short time in the summer months and expose their forearms, hands and face to the sun. For those who do not have the benefit of sunlight because they are completely housebound or do not wish to remove enveloping clothes, a good dietary source of vitamin D such as margarine, eggs or oily fish (e.g. sardines, mackerel) is important, and they should preferably take an additional supplement of 10 µg of vitamin D each day. The importance of vitamin D and calcium for healthy bones is widely recognised but other nutrients have been identified as being important for bones – many of these nutrients are found in fruits and vegetables. Several studies have shown that fruit and vegetable consumption is associated with a decrease in the risk of fracture. There is some evidence to suggest that high intakes of vitamin A may increase the risk of bone fracture. Liver is a rich source of vitamin A, so older people should avoid eating liver or liver products such as pâté more than once a week, or should eat smaller portions. If they do eat liver once a week they should avoid taking any supplements containing vitamin A or fish liver oils (which contain high levels of vitamin A). Experts recommend that older people at risk of osteoporosis should not consume more than 1500 µg (1.5 mg) of vitamin A per day from diet and supplements combined.

Slimmers

Energy needs and food consumption have been discussed in Chapter 5. Planning a slimming diet is a matter of individual preference. Essentially, the energy intake needs to be cut down by 2 - 4 MJ (500 - 1000 kcal) each day to achieve a weekly weight loss of 0.5 - 1.0 kg (1-2 lb). Other nutrients should still reach recommended levels. It is often convenient to cut out fatty and sugary foods such as cakes, sweets, preserves, biscuits and some puddings as well as alcohol, as these tend to be sources of energy rather than nutrients. Low- or reduced-fat and sugar products, now readily available, can be substituted for traditionally high-fat and sugar foods. Fat can be trimmed from meat, and foods can be boiled or grilled and not fried. Foods high in water or fibre can induce feelings of fullness and so help to reduce the desire for more food.

Effective slimming diets are all basically low energy or 'low calorie' diets, though they vary in how this is achieved. A good plan is to base meals on a modest helping of lean meat, fish, eggs or reduced-fat cheese with liberal amounts of fruits and vegetables and moderate amounts of bread, potatoes, rice and pasta. Eating three or four meals a day gives better results than eating the same amount of food at one or two meals only. Including breakfast, ideally based on a whole-grain breakfast cereal with skimmed milk or yogurt and fruit, helps to avoid mid-morning hunger. As it may take several months to reach the desired healthy weight, a slimming diet should be sensible and palatable enough to be tolerated for this length of time. After this, it is advisable to keep to the changes made to the diet whilst slimming and gradually increase the energy content until the new healthy weight is maintained. Diets which cut out whole food groups are not recommended. There is insufficient evidence to say whether such diets are free from negative health effects or that they are effective and achieve sustainable weight loss. Diets based on only one or two foods may be successful in the short term but are hard to adhere to as they are unrealistic, dull, and do not teach healthy eating habits; they can also be deficient in a range of nutrients and therefore dangerous. Very-low-calorie diets (VLCDs) (less than 3.4 MJ (800 kcal) per day) are unsuitable for infants, children, adolescents, pregnant or lactating women, the elderly and people with certain medical conditions, e.g. heart disease.

There are times when it is difficult to reduce food intake especially on social occasions but by planning to eat less for a day or two beforehand, it is possible to enjoy food on such occasions without weight gain. Keeping to a slimming diet can sometimes be made easier by joining a slimmers' group, and weight loss is improved by being physically active.

Vegetarians

Most vegetarians are lacto-ovo vegetarians and do not eat meat, fish, seafood or by-products of animal slaughter such as gelatine, but will eat milk, cheese and eggs. Such diets may be rather bulky and lower in energy than a mixed diet because most vegetables have a high water content but, in general, their nutritional values are very similar to those of mixed diets.

A much smaller group, *vegans*, eats no foods of animal origin at all. Human nutrient requirements, with the exception of vitamin B_{12} (p. 66), can be met by a diet composed entirely of plant foods, but to do so it must be carefully planned using a wide selection of foods. A mixture of plant proteins derived from cereals, peas, beans and nuts will provide enough protein of good quality, but special care is needed to ensure that sufficient energy, calcium, iron, riboflavin, vitamin B_{12} and vitamin D are also available. Yeast extract is a good source of some of the B-vitamins including vitamin B_{12} which are otherwise found mainly in foods of animal origin. In extreme cases, such as Zen macrobiotic diets where little but whole-grain cereals are eaten, intakes of calcium, iron, vitamin B_{12} and vitamin C are likely to be too low for health.

Some people, both vegetarian and non-vegetarian, prefer to eat only or mainly 'organic' foods. All foods, being derived from plants or animals, are organic; and all foods because they provide nutrients, are conducive to health when eaten as part of a balanced diet as described in this manual. The word 'organic' has, however, come to acquire the restricted meaning of foods grown without the use of inorganic fertilisers, pesticides or herbicides, and either not processed or processed without the use of additives. The use of additives aids the production and economic distribution of the food needed for our dense urban population and is controlled by legislation (p. 166). On the basis of current evidence there is no significant difference between organic and conventionally produced food in terms of nutrition (or food safety).

Ethnic groups

In general the traditional diets of ethnic communities provide adequate nourishment to those who consume them. Recent immigrants to the UK, who have difficulty adapting their traditional diets and customs (see Table 35) to local circumstances, may have special dietary problems. In particular, Asian vegetarian groups may have very low intakes of vitamin D. As exposure to sunlight (especially by women and children) may also be low due to customs of dress and because they tend to remain indoors, rickets and osteomalacia sometimes develop. Good sources of vitamin D should therefore be included in sufficient quantity in the diet and vitamin supplements may be necessary. Iron deficiency anaemia sometimes occurs among women and children, particularly in the Asian community, since the iron content of certain traditional diets may also be low.

Some ethnic minorities appear to be at much greater risk of chronic diseases such as diabetes, coronary heart disease, stroke and hypertension than the general UK population. This is a result of a complex interplay of many factors, of which diet, like physical activity, is modifiable and therefore healthy eating messages may be particularly pertinent to these groups.

Diabetics

Diabetes is a metabolic disorder, which reduces the ability of the body to control the amount of glucose in the blood. It is important for diabetics to avoid the large rises in blood glucose that can result from eating readily absorbed carbohydrate, but this requires control rather than a reduction in total carbohydrate intake. Indeed, many Asian diabetics live well with 60 per cent or more of their diet as carbohydrate from rice or chapatis, whereas traditional low-carbohydrate diets, being high in saturated fat, may have contributed to the prevalence of heart disease in British diabetics.

Table 35. Dietary restrictions practiced by religious and ethnic groups

Hindus	No beef	Mostly vegetarian; fish rarely eaten; no alcohol	Period of fasting common
Muslim	No pork	Meat must be 'Halal'; no shellfish eaten; no alcohol	Regular fasting, including Ramadan for one month
Sikhs	No beef	Meat must be killed by, one blow to the head'; no alcohol	Generally less rigid eating restrictions than Hindus and Muslims
Jews	No pork	Meat must be kosher; only fish with scales and fins eaten	Meat and dairy foods must not be consumed together
Rastafarians	No animal products except milk may be consumed	Foods must be 'I-tal' or alive, so no canned or processed foods eaten; no salt added; no coffee or alcohol	Food should be organic

Halal meat is dedicated to God by a Muslim present at the killing. Kosher meat must be slaughtered by a Rabbinical-licensed person and then soaked and salted

Glycaemic Index

The Glycaemic Index (GI) ranks carbohydrate-containing foods based on their potential to raise blood glucose. Carbohydrates that are rapidly broken down cause a rapid increase in blood glucose and have a high GI rating. High GI foods include sugar and sugary foods, soft drinks, white bread, potatoes, white rice etc. Low or medium GI foods include fruits and vegetables that have not been dried, pulses and whole grain foods. Protein and fat slows down the absorption of carbohydrate and mixing high GI foods with foods with low GI will give a meal with a medium GI. It is useful for diabetics to understand the concept of GI so that they can consume high GI foods with care and avoid consuming these foods alone. However, diabetics are advised to eat a healthy, balanced diet as recommended for the population in general.

It is particularly important for diabetics to control their weight since obesity can worsen diabetic control.

Other special diets

The principles set out in this manual hold in general for all healthy individuals. There are, however, some people who are allergic or intolerant to certain foods, for example peanuts, nuts, milk, eggs, shellfish or wheat gluten. Allergic reactions to such foods can result in the rapid onset of anaphylactic shock which, unless treated immediately, can be fatal. People with conditions such as coeliac disease (p. 22) or lactose intolerance (p. 6) also need to avoid any foods containing gluten or milk, respectively.

Such intolerances are not normally life threatening and the amounts of the foods that can be consumed without adverse effect will vary from person to person. When certain drugs are taken, the avoidance of specific foods (e.g. cheese) is necessary. These allergies and illnesses are a medical rather than a nutritional problem.

Summary: assessing the adequacy of a diet

It is important not only that all the essential nutrients should be present in the foods eaten, but also that they should be present in the amounts required by different people. To find out whether a particular diet is nutritionally adequate, three things must be known:

(a) What foods were eaten?
(b) How much of each food was eaten?
(c) What kind of person or people ate the foods? Were they men, women, adolescents or children, and were they very active or sedentary? Were any of the women pregnant or breast-feeding a baby?

When the answers to these questions are known, daily nutrient intakes can then be compared with the Dietary Reference Values and any other appropriate guidelines. It must, however, be emphasised that the RNIs for minerals and vitamins are high enough to cover the needs of practically all healthy people; someone who obtains less than the RNI is not necessarily deficient in that nutrient. An individual will only give cause for concern if they are consistently obtaining less than the LRNI.

Four important methods of measuring food consumption are:

(a) Measuring the amount of food and drink purchased both for the home and for eating outside the home by, for example, a family over one or two weeks. Surveys of food purchases at the household level, such as the UK Expenditure and Food Survey[4], provide estimates of population average food consumption, based on purchase information and the number of people in each household. It is important to note that this type of survey does not measure what individuals actually eat and may not take account of wastage.
(b) Recalling, preferably with expert help, all the foods eaten in the previous 24 hours. This is the least time-consuming method, but it is easy to forget important foods and hard to estimate quantities accurately. Repeated 24-hour recalls may be used to get a better picture of usual diet. This method may be supplemented with a diet history that records a person's recollection of their 'typical' 7-day eating pattern.

---

[4] The Expenditure and Food Survey is a survey of household food purchases and food eaten outside the home that provides annual trend data on food expenditure, consumption and nutrient intakes at the population level. The EFS replaced the long running National Food Survey in 2001. Over 6000 households in the UK take part each year by recording purchases of household food and food eaten outside the home for a 2-week period. The survey provides population average data on food consumption, expenditure and nutrient intake at the household level. Results can be broken down into various household characteristics such as region or income group.

(c) Recording details of (and sometimes weighing) all the foods eaten or drunk over a specified period (usually a week). Provided that the diet is not changed to accommodate the complex recording procedure, this should be the most precise method of assessing the value of anyone's diet. However, some people may, consciously or otherwise, make alterations to their normal diet during the survey week or omit to report some foods that were eaten. This method was used for the National Diet and Nutrition Survey[5] of adults aged 19 to 64, which furnished the nutrient intake data quoted throughout this Manual, and for the National Diet and Nutrition Surveys of other population groups referred to in Appendix 9.

(d) Responding to a food frequency questionnaire to say how often each food from a list is eaten in terms of x times per day/per week/per month. It may also include assessment of the quantity of food consumed on each eating occasion. A limited range of foods may be singled out for study if it is not necessary to assess the total diet. Food frequency questionnaires are quick and easy to complete, but do not provide precise estimates of food consumption.

It is easy to determine the weights of standard or pre-packaged items, and for meals served in some canteens or restaurants it may be possible to weigh all the components of duplicates of the meal. More care is needed to evaluate variable items such as stews in either the domestic or catering contexts. It is also important to remember that the nutrient content of foods may vary from the average values shown in this manual.

As an example of the way in which a diet can be evaluated, the daily pattern of snacks and meals, which might have been eaten by a young man in a sedentary occupation, has been set out in a systematic way in Table 36. The nutrients provided by these quantities of each of these foods must be calculated using food tables such as that in Appendix 3. The results can be summarised meal by meal as in Table 37, or the contribution of each food to each nutrient can be listed if the evaluation covers only a short period.

---

[5] The National Diet and Nutrition Surveys constitute a programme of national surveys of various population groups with the aim of gathering information about the dietary habits and nutritional status of the British population. The results of these surveys are used to develop national nutrition policy and contribute to the evidence base for Government advice on healthy eating.

Table 36. Menu for one day for a young sedentary man

	Weight (g)		Weight (g)
Breakfast		*Evening meal*	
Orange juice, unsweetened	150	Spaghetti	230
Cornflakes	50	Bolognese sauce	240
Milk, semi-skimmed	146	Cheddar cheese	20
Sugar with cornflakes	10	Ice cream, dairy, vanilla	75
White bread, 2 slices, toasted	54	Peaches, canned in syrup	120
Fat spread (70-80% fat, blended)	18		
Marmalade	30		
1 cup of tea			
Milk, semi-skimmed with tea	30		
Sugar with tea	10		
Lunch (sandwich)		*Snacks throughout the day*	
White baguette	120	2 cups of coffee	
Fat spread (70-80% fat, blended)	20	Milk, semi-skimmed with coffee	60
Tuna, canned in brine	45	Sugar with coffee	20
Mayonnaise	15	1 packet crisps	35
Banana	100	1 apple	100
1 can of carbonated drink		Chocolate bar	66
(cola, non-diet)	343		
		1 pint lager	574

The intakes of nutrients can then be compared with the Dietary Reference Values for such a person, and with an understanding of the principles set out in this manual the significance of any departures from these values can be assessed. In the instance of the menu for this particular man (as seen in Table 37):

Calcium, iron, folate and vitamin C intakes are well above the RNIs for these nutrients. In general it is easier for men to achieve these levels than women because they eat larger quantities of food. The *sodium* content of the day's meals is more than twice the suggested RNI for an adult. This equates to about 9 g salt and is much higher than SACN recommended maximum daily adult intake of 6 g per day. It would be advisable for this young man to moderate his salt intake by, for example, substituting a lower-sodium cereal for cornflakes, replacing a salty snack like crisps with a low-fat yogurt or fruit, and adding less salt to the main dish during cooking.

The *energy* intake is a little higher than the EAR for a man aged between 19 and 40 with a physical activity level of 1.4. Many sedentary men have lower energy intakes than this, and it is possible that this young man could gain weight if such a meal pattern were eaten regularly. The proportion of total energy derived from *protein* is 11.3 %, which is acceptable. The proportion of the total energy intake derived from *fat* is 33.3 %, from *saturated fat* 13.7 % and from *carbohydrate* 50.6 %. If the total fat intake was maintained at or about this level over the course of time, the fat content of the whole diet would be very satisfactory. The percentage of energy from saturated fat Is above the recommended 10% of food energy. If this higher intake of saturated fat was maintained then it could have a detrimental effect on blood cholesterol and, over time, increase this man's risk of heart disease. Eating lean meat or fish without a cheese sauce and accompanied by a baked potato, with a little low fat spread, and vegetables for the evening meal would be one way of reducing his intake of saturated fatty acids. If he wished to treat himself to a chocolate bar on another day he might want to substitute low-fat yogurt for ice cream in the evening and fresh fruit or salad items for the crisps or biscuits during snack times. An increase in his intake of starch-rich foods at the expense of sugar could improve his intake of *fibre* as NSP (which is a little low), especially if whole-grain products are consumed. Alternatively, it could be raised by, for example, substituting a high-fibre cereal for cornflakes at breakfast.

It should be recalled that the DRVs for fat, saturated fatty acids and carbohydrate are meant to be applied to populations of people rather than individuals. Therefore it is desirable for a group of men of this age and lifestyle who, as individuals, vary in their nutrient needs, to consume on average over time a diet which achieves the DRVs, rather than each individual aiming to achieve the DRVs every day. Nevertheless, if each individual tries to make changes towards a more healthy diet, the more likelihood there is that the population as a whole will achieve the DRVs.[6]

---

[6] To help people to attain a sensible balance and variety of foods for a healthy diet, the UK Government has apportioned foods into five groups, namely bread, rice, potatoes, pasta and other starchy foods, fruit and vegetables, meat, fish, eggs, beans and other non-dairy sources of protein, milk and dairy foods and food and drinks high in fat and/or sugar. The proportions in which these food groups should be eaten for a healthy, balanced diet are shown in the Eatwell plate in Appendix 6.

Table 37. Nutrient content of a day's menu for a young sedentary man

	Energy (kJ)	Energy (kcal)	Protein (g)	Fat (g)	Saturated fat (g)	Carbo-hydrate (g)	Fibre (g)	Calcium (mg)	Iron (mg)	Sodium (mg)	Folate (µg)	Vitamin C (mg)
Breakfast	3209	767	16.1	18.0	6.9	144.1	1.9	358	5.4	1015	222	63
Lunch	3494	835	22.9	29.1	7.4	128.4	4.0	179	2.5	1103	51	11
Evening meal	3799	908	45.0	43.8	19.2	88.7	5.3	281	4.0	929	57	14
Snacks	3552	849	11.2	33.4	17.6	91.8	4.2	262	1.6	406	91	19
Total	14054	3359	95.2	124.3	51.1	453.0	15.4	1080	12.9	3453	421	107
			11.3[a]	33.3[a]	13.7[a]	50.6[a]						
EAR (DH 1991)	10600	2550	44.4	33[a]	10[a]	47[a]	18	525	6.7		150	25
RNI (DH 1991)			55.5					700	8.7	1600	200	40
LRNI (DH 1991)								400	4.7	575	100	10

[a] As a percentage of total energy.
See also Table 33.

APPENDICES

Appendix 1 Common Measure and conversion factors

Although the labels of most pre-packed foods give their weight in grams, many fresh foods are weighed in imperial units and many individuals still use pounds (weight), pints, inches, etc. Furthermore energy has long been measured in calories, but the SI units joules are also being used. The conversion

Weight

1 milligram (mg)	= 1000 micrograms (μg)	
1 gram (g)	= 1000 mg	= 0.035 oz
1 kilogram (kg)	= 1000 g	= 2.20 lb
1 ounce (oz)	= 28.35 g	
1 pound (lb)	= 453.6 g	

Volume

1 litre	= 1000 millilitres (ml)	= 1.76 pt
1 pint (pt	= 20 fluid oz	= 568 ml

Length

1 metre (m)	= 100 centimetres (cm)	= 1000 milimetres (mm)
		= 39.4 in
1 inch (in)	= 2.54 cm	
1 foot (ft)	= 0.3048 m	

Energy

1 kilojoule (kJ)	= 1000 joules (J)	
1 megajoule (MJ)	= 1000 kJ	= 239 kcal
1 kilocalorie (kcal)	= 41.184 kJ	

Appendix 2   Equations for estimating the basal metabolic rate (BMR)

BMR (MJ/day)

Males	10-17 years	BMR = 0.074W + 2.754
	18-29 years	BMR = 0.063W + 2.896
	30-59 years	BMR = 0.048W + 3.653
	Over 60 years	BMR = 0.049W + 2.459
Females	10-17 years	BMR = 0.056W + 2.898
	18-29 years	BMR = 0.062W + 2.036
	30-59 years	BMR = 0.034W + 3.538
	Over 60 years	BMR = 0.038W + 2.755

BMR (kcal/day)

Males.	10-17 years	BMR = 17.7W + 657
	18-29 years	BMR = 15.1 W + 692
	30-59 years	BMR = 11.5W + 873
Females	10-17 years	BMR = 13.4W + 692
	18-29 years	BMR = 14.8W + 487
	30-59 years	BMR = 8.3W + 846

W = body weight (kg)

Example: A woman, 40 years old, who weighs 62kg

$$BMR = (0.034 \times 62) + 3.538$$
$$= 2.108 + 3.538 = 5.646$$
$$= 5.7 \text{ MJ/day}$$

or $BMR = (8.3 \times 62) + 846 = 515 + 846$
$$= 1361 \text{ kcal/day}$$

Appendix 3   Composition of food

Typical values for the amounts of a number of nutrients in a wide variety of raw and cooked foods are shown in the following table. Each value is the amount per 100 g of the edible part of the food as described. The information is based on the sixth summary edition of *McCance and Widdowson's The Composition of Foods* (2002), which gives details of more foods and more nutrients than are shown here. Individual samples of food can differ considerably depending on the season of the year; therefore, any information given on the label by the manufacturers should be more appropriate for that particular product than the more general values in this Appendix.

Allowance may need to be made for wastage in foods that are weighed raw. The values given here predict the proportion of each food as listed that cannot be eaten. Thus for raw chicken it is the amount of skin and bone likely to be in the whole or joint of a chicken to be cooked, but for slices of roast chicken there would be no wastage. Some individuals may, however, choose not to eat some of the fat or to discard any parts of a fruit that are bruised, and an additional allowance may have to be made for this.

The energy value of each food is given in kilojoules (kJ) and kilocalories (kcal), and both have been calculated from the protein, fat and carbohydrate content as on p. 32. The figures for vitamin A are given in the form of retinol equivalents (p. 58). They are thus expressed in the same form as in the *Dietary Reference Values for Food Energy and Nutrients for the United Kingdom* (1991). Available carbohydrate is given as its monosaccharide equivalent (p. 9). Appendix 4 provides examples of the use of this table.

Table 3.1 Composition per 100 g of edible portion

No.	Food	Inedible waste (%)	Water (g) (mg)	Energy (kj)	Energy kcal	Protein (g)	Fat (g)	Saturated Fatty Acid (g)
	Cereals							
1	Flour, plain, white	0	14.0	1450	341	9.4	1.3	0.2
2	Flour, wholemeal	0	14.0	1318	310	12.7	2.2	0.3
3	Brown rice, boiled	0	66.0	597	141	2.6	1.1	0.3
4	White rice, easy cook, boiled	0	68.0	587	138	2.6	1.3	0.3
5	Spaghetti, white, boiled	0	73.8	442	104	3.6	0.7	0.1
6	Pizza, cheese and tomato, thin base	0	40.6	1168	277	14.4	10.3	4.8
7	Pasta, plain, fresh, cooked	0	61.5	677	159	6.6	1.5	0.3
8	Pasta, fresh, cheese and vegetable stuffed, cooked	1	61.3	714	169	7.7	4.6	N
	Breads							
9	Brown bread, average	0	41.2	882	207	7.9	2.0	0.4
10	White bread, sliced	0	38.6	931	219	7.9	1.6	0.3
11	White bread, 'with added fibre'	0	40.0	978	230	7.6	1.5	0.4
12	Ciabatta	0	29.2	1150	271	10.2	3.9	0.6
13	Wholemeal bread, average	0	41.2	922	217	9.4	2.5	0.5
14	Granary bread	0	34.9	1005	237	9.6	2.3	0.6
	Breakfast cereals							
15	Bran Flakes	0	3.0	1406	330	10.2	2.5	0.4
16	Corn Flakes	0	3.0	1601	376	7.9	0.9	0.2
17	Muesli, Swiss style	0	7.2	1540	363	9.8	5.9	0.8
18	Weetabix	0	5.6	1498	352	11.2	2.7	0.6
19	Frosties	0	3.0	1626	381	5.3	0.6	0.1
20	Porridge, made with whole milk	0	74.8	472	113	4.8	5.1	2.8
	Biscuits							
21	Chocolate biscuits, full coated	0	1.2	2105	501	7.3	24.3	13.2
22	Cream crackers	0	4.3	1746	414	9.5	13.3	5.4
23	Digestive biscuits, plain	0	2.5	1956	465	6.3	20.3	9.0
24	Semi-sweet biscuits	0	2.5	1803	427	6.7	13.3	6.3
	Buns and cakes							
25	Currant buns	0	27.9	1185	280	8.0	5.6	1.9
26	Fruit cake, rich	0	17.5	1447	343	3.9	11.4	2.4
27	Flapjack	0	6.6	2064	493	4.8	27.0	4.9
28	Gateau, fruit, frozen	0	51.9	1042	248	3.2	12.3	7.0
29	Madeira cake	0	20.2	1585	377	5.4	15.1	8.4
30	Muffins, American style, chocolate chip	0	22.3	1617	385	6.3	18.2	10.7
31	Swiss roll, chocolate, individual	0	17.5	1624	386	4.3	16.8	7.0
	Puddings and Dairy Desserts							
32	Crumble, fruit	0	49.1	924	219	2.4	8.3	4.0

Carbo-hydrate (g)	Total Sugars (g)	Fibre NSP (g)	Calcium (mg)	Iron (mg)	Sodium (mg)	Vitamin A (µg)	Folate (µg)	Vitamin C (mg)	No.
77.7	1.5	3.1	140	2.0	3	0	??	0	1
63.9	2.1	9.0	30	3.9	3	0	57	0	2
32.1	0.5	0.8	4	0.5	1	0	10	0	3
30.9	0.0	0.1	18	0.2	1	0	7	0	4
22.2	0.5	1.2	7	0.5	0	0	7	0	5
33.9	2.5	1.9	279	1.1	282	80	7	1	6
31.8	0.6	1.9	37	0.8	16	0	4	0	7
25.8	0.9	1.3	115	0.9	204	25	3	0	8
42.1	3.4	3.5	186	2.2	443	0	45	0	9
46.1	3.4	1.9	177	1.6	461	0	25	0	10
49.6	3.3	3.1	150	2.3	450	0	(17)	0	11
52.0	3.1	2.3	(121)	(1.4)	538	0	21	0	12
42.0	2.8	5.0	106	2.4	487	0	40	0	13
47.4	2.9	3.3	209	1.9	545	0	88	0	14
71.2	22.8	13.0	40	24.3	800	0	333	66	15
89.6	8.2	0.9	5	7.9	1000	0	333	0	16
72.2	26.2	6.4	110	5.8	380	0	(140)	0	17
75.5	4.9	9.7	35	11.9	270	0	170	0	18
94.6	44	0.6	453	7.9	600	0	167	0	19
12.6	4.8	0.9	128	0.5	595	37	10	1	20
67.6	45.8	1.5	130	1.3	235	27	9	0	21
68.3	0.0	2.2	110	1.7	610	0	(22)	0	22
60.6	13.6	2.2	92	3.2	600	0	13	0	23
74.8	22.3	1.7	120	2.1	410	0	(13)	0	24
52.6	16.0	2.2	110	1.9	317	0	12	1	25
59.9	48.7	1.5	79	2.1	155	109	8	0	26
62.4	34.5	2.6	36	2.3	264	210	11	0	27
33.3	14.9	0.9	40	0.7	128	118	6	4	28
58.4	36.5	0.9	42	1.1	380	N	N	0	29
52.3	28.4	1.6	161	1.45	254	144	10	0	30
58.1	41.8	N	77	1.1	350	N	10	0	31
36.0	22.0	1.3	41	0.3	82	53	10	N	32

Table 3.1 Composition per 100 g of edible portion (continued).

No.	Food	Inedible waste (%)	Water (g)	Energy (kj)	kcal	Protein (g)	Fat (g)	Saturated Fatty Acid (g)
33	Fruit pie, pastry top and bottom	0	47.8	1096	262	3.1	13.6	4.2
34	Cheesecake, fruit, individual	0	46.6	1111	264	6.1	12.3	7.5
35	Custard, made up with semi-skimmed milk	0	77.5	404	95	4.0	2.0	1.2
36	Rice pudding, canned	0	79.2	362	85	3.3	1.3	0.8
37	Trifle	0	66.5	696	166	2.6	8.1	2.4
38	Lemon meringue pie	0	42.1	1060	251	2.9	8.5	3.1
39	Mousse, chocolate	0	67.3	627	149	4.0	6.5	3.3
40	Mousse, chocolate, reduced fat	0	69.0	518	123	5.5	3.7	2.5
41	Ice-cream, dairy, premium	0	60.9	894	215	3.9	15.1	9.1
42	Ice-cream, non-dairy, vanilla	0	66.5	640	153	3.0	7.8	4.8
	Milk and cream							
43	Skimmed milk, average	0	90.9	136	32	3.4	0.2	0.1
44	Semi-skimmed milk, average	0	89.6	195	46	3.4	1.7	1.1
45	Whole milk, average	0	87.6	274	66	3.3	3.9	2.5
46	Dried skimmed milk	0	3.0	1482	348	36.1	0.6	0.4
47	Cream, single	0	77.0	798	193	3.3	19.1	12.2
48	Cream, double	0	46.9	2041	496	1.6	53.7	33.4
	Yoghurt and Fromage Frais							
49	Whole milk yogurt, plain	0	81.9	333	79	5.7	3.0	1.7
	Whole milk yoghurt, twinpot, thick and creamy, with fruit	0	74.7	446	106	4.1	3.2	N
50	Low fat yoghurt, fruit	0	78.9	331	78	4.2	1.1	(0.8)
51	Virtually fat free/diet yoghurt, fruit	0	85.4	201	47	4.8	0.2	(0.1)
52	Fromage frais, fruit	0	74.7	520	124	5.3	5.6	3.5
53	Milkshake, thick, takeaway	0	73.2	374	88	3.7	1.8	1.2
	Cheese							
54	Brie	31	48.7	1422	343	20.3	29.1	18.2
55	Cheddar cheese	0	36.6	1725	416	25.4	34.9	21.7
56	Cheddar type, half fat	0	47.4	1141	273	32.7	15.8	9.9
57	Cheese spread, plain	0	58.8	1106	267	11.3	22.8	15.8
58	Spreadable cheese, soft white, full fat	0	58.6	1286	312	7.5	31.3	20.5
59	Cottage cheese, plain	0	78.6	423	101	12.6	4.3	2.3
60	Feta	0	56.5	1037	250	15.6	20.2	(13.7)
61	Mozzarella, fresh	0	57.4	1067	257	18.6	20.3	13.8
62	Processed cheese, plain	0	47.4	1234	297	17.8	23.0	14.3
63	Stilton, blue	0	38.0	1698	410	23.7	35.0	23.0
	Eggs							
64	Eggs, chicken, boiled	0	75.1	612	147	12.5	10.8	3.1
65	Eggs, chicken, fried in vegetable oil	0	70.1	745	179	13.6	13.9	4.0

Carbo-hydrate (g)	Total Sugars (g)	Fibre NSP (g)	Calcium (mg)	Iron (mg)	Sodium (mg)	Vitamin A (µg)	Folate (µg)	Vitamin C (mg)	No.
33.9	12.0	1.7	58	0.8	193	65	7	3	33
34.5	25.4	1.0	78	0.4	151	N	(7)	U	34
16.4	11.3	0.0	140	0.1	67	98	6	1	35
16.1	8.7	0.1	88	0.1	43	18	0	0	36
21.0	16.7	0.4	57	0.3	70	118	6	5	37
43.5	29.8	(0.7)	38	0.0	113	48	6	5	38
19.9	17.5	N	97	0.2	67	48	6	0	39
18.0	15.8	N	126	1.2	69	N	0	0	40
16.7	16.7	0.0	(100)	0.0	(60)	177	(6)	(1)	41
18.0	18.0	0.0	72	0.1	62	2	8	1	42
4.4	4.4	0.0	122	0.03	44	1	9	1	43
4.7	4.7	0.0	120	0.02	43	21	6	1	44
4.5	4.5	0.0	118	0.03	43	36	8	2	45
52.9	52.9	0.0	1280	0.27	550	351	51	13	46
2.2	2.2	0.0	89	0.0	29	319	5	1	47
1.7	1.7	0.0	49	0.1	22	860	7	1	48
7.8	7.8	N	200	0.1	80	28	18	1	49
16.2	15.6	N	130	0.2	53	(20)	(13)	(2)	
13.7	12.7	0.2	140	0.1	62	(10)	16	1	50
7.0	6.3	0.0	130	0.1	73	0	8	1	51
13.9	13.3	0.0	86	0.1	35	82	15	0	52
15.3	11.1	0.0	129	0.0	57	35	4	1	53
0.0	0.0	0.0	256	0.0	556	329	55	0	54
0.1	0.1	0.0	739	0.3	723	388	31	0	55
0.0	0.0	0.0	840	0.2	670	210	56	0	56
4.4	4.4	0.0	498	0.0	1077	282	19	0	57
0.0	0.0	0.0	76	0.0	288	293	23	0	58
3.1	3.1	0.0	(127)	0.0	(300)	48	(22)	0	59
1.5	1.5	0.0	360	0.2	1440	226	23	0	60
0.0	0.0	0.0	362	0.0	395	283	20	0	61
5.0	5.0	0.0	610	0.5	1351	286	15	0	62
0.1	0.1	0.0	326	0.2	788	390	78	0	63
0.0	0.0	0.0	57	1.9	140	190	39	0	64
0.0	0.0	0.0	65	2.2	160	215	40	0	65

Table 3.1 Composition per 100 g of edible portion (continued).

No.	Food	Inedible waste (%)	Water (g) (mg)	Energy (kj)	Energy kcal	Protein (g)	Fat (g)	Saturated Fatty Acid (g)
	Fats and oils							
66	Butter	0	14.9	3059	744	0.6	82.2	52.1
67	Margarine, soft, polyunsaturated	0	16.0	3067	746	0.0	82.8	17.0
68	Fat spread (60% fat), polyunsaturated	0	(37.7)	2274	553	0.2	60.8	11.3
69	(35-40% fat), polyunsaturated	0	53.8	1503	365	4.9	37.6	8.9
70	Blended spread (70-80% fat)	0	21.0	2795	680	0.6	74.8	25.5
71	Sunflower oil	0	0.0	3696	899	0.0	99.9	12.0
72	Vegetable oil, blended, average	0	0.0	3696	899	0.0	99.9	11.7
73	Olive oil	0	0.0	3696	899	0.0	99.9	14.3
	Meat and meat products							
74	Bacon rasher, lean and fat, grilled, back	0	50.4	1194	287	23.2	21.6	8.1
75	Bacon rasher, lean and fat, grilled, streaky	0	44.0	1400	337	23.8	26.9	9.8
76	Beef, mince, stewed	0	64.4	870	209	21.8	13.5	5.7
77	Beef, mince, extra lean, stewed	0	66.6	742	177	24.7	8.7	3.8
78	Beef, stewing steak, lean and fat, stewed	0	59.4	852	203	29.2	9.6	3.7
79	Beef, rump steak, fried, lean	0	61.7	770	183	30.9	6.6	2.4
80	Beef burgers, frozen, grilled	0	47.9	1355	326	26.5	24.4	10.9
81	Bolognese sauce, with meat	0	70.8	670	161	11.8	11.6	4.2
82	Chicken, roast, meat average	0	65.3	742	177	27.3	7.5	2.9
83	Chicken skin	0	31.1	2070	501	21.5	46.1	12.9
84	Chicken, stir fried strips	0	65.9	677	161	29.7	4.6	N
85	Corned beef, canned	0	59.5	860	205	25.9	10.9	5.7
86	Ham, sliced	0	73.2	451	107	18.4	3.3	1.1
87	Kidney, pig, stewed	0	66.3	641	153	24.4	6.1	2.0
88	Lamb, roast, lean	0	54.4	1138	273	26.7	18.5	8.6
89	Lamb, loin chops, grilled, meat only	39	59.6	892	213	29.2	10.7	4.9
90	Liver, lamb, fried	0	53.9	989	237	30.1	12.9	N
91	Pate, liver	0	47.6	1437	348	12.6	32.7	9.5
92	Pork, loin chops, lean only, grilled	23	61.2	774	184	31.6	6.4	2.2
93	Pork, leg joint, roasted medium, lean	15	61.1	765	182	33.0	5.5	1.9
94	Salami	0	33.7	1814	438	20.9	39.2	14.6
95	Sausages, beef, grilled	0	48.0	1157	278	13.3	19.5	7.9
96	Sausages, pork grilled	0	45.9	1221	294	14.5	22.1	8.0
97	Sausages, low fat, grilled	0	50.1	959	230	16.2	13.8	4.9
98	Steak and kidney/beef pie, individual, baked	0	41.4	1295	310	8.8	19.4	8.4
99	Turkey, roast, meat only	0	64.6	701	166	31.2	4.6	1.4
100	Lasagne, chilled/frozen, reheated	0	68.1	603	143	7.4	6.1	2.8
101	Chicken curry, average	0	70.2	603	145	11.7	9.8	2.9
102	Chicken nuggets	0	47.8	1111	265	18.7	13.0	3.3

Carbo-hydrate (g)	Total Sugars (g)	Fibre NSP (g)	Calcium (mg)	Iron (mg)	Sodium (mg)	Vitamin A (µg)	Folate (µg)	Vitamin C (mg)	No.
0.6	0.6	0.0	18	0.0	606	1059	0	0	66
0.2	0.2	0.0	1	0.3	680	733	0	0	67
1.3	1.3	0.0	N	0.0	710	980	0	0	68
1.8	1.3	0.0	N	0.0	650	N	0	0	69
1.1	1.1	0.0	14	0.0	670	565	0	0	70
0.0	0.0	0.0	0	0.1	0	0	0	0	71
0.0	0.0	0.0	0	0.0	0	0	0	0	72
0.0	0.0	0.0	0	0.4	0	0	0	0	73
0.0	0.0	0.0	7	0.6	1880	0	5	0	74
0.0	0.0	0.0	9	0.8	1680	0	3	0	75
0.0	0.0	0.0	20	2.7	73	13	17	0	76
0.0	0.0	0.0	14	2.3	75	1	20	0	77
0.0	0.0	0.0	15	2.3	51	1	11	0	78
0.0	0.0	0.0	5	3.0	78	1	5	0	79
0.1	0.1	0.0	10	2.5	400	0	10	0	80
2.5	2.1	0.6	16	1.06	306	123	9	3	81
0.0	0.0	0.0	17	0.8	100	24	10	0	82
0.0	0.0	0.0	16	1.3	80	N	N	0	83
0.0	0.0	0.0	6	0.5	61	0	5	0	84
1.0	1.0	0.0	27	2.4	860	0	5	0	85
1.0	1.00	0.0	7	0.7	1200	0	19	0	86
0.0	0.0	0.0	13	6.4	370	46	43	11	87
0.0	0.0	0.0	8	1.6	93	0	6	0	88
0.0	0.0	0.0	22	2.1	80	0	6	0	89
0.0	0.0	0.0	8	7.7	82	(1910)	207	19	90
(0.8)	0.4	0.0	16	5.9	750	7322	99	N	91
0.0	0.0	0.0	14	0.7	66	0	7	0	92
0.0	0.0	0.0	10	1.1	69	0	4	0	93
0.5	0.5	0.1	11	1.3	1800	0	3	N	94
13.1	1.4	0.7	80	1.4	1200	0	7	N	95
9.8	1.5	0.7	110	1.1	1080	0	4	5	96
10.8	0.9	1.5	130	1.3	1180	0	32	37	97
26.7	1.5	0.5	60	1.3	460	8	(8)	0	98
0.0	0.0	0.0	11	0.8	90	0	17	0	99
15.7	3.0	0.7	80	1.0	390	N	11	N	100
2.5	1.2	2.0	41	2.32	356	35	N	0	101
19.5	1.1	0.2	25	0.6	510	14	20	0	102

149

Table 3.1 Composition per 100 g of edible portion (continued).

No.	Food	Inedible waste (%)	Water (g) (mg)	Energy (kj)	kcal	Protein (g)	Fat (g)	Saturated Fatty Acids (g)
	Fish and Fish Products							
103	Cod in batter, fried in blended oil	0	54.9	1031	247	16.1	15.4	1.6
104	Fish fingers, grilled	0	55.7	838	200	14.3	8.9	2.8
105	Haddock, steamed, flesh only	16	78.3	378	89	20.9	0.6	0.1
106	Mackerel, grilled	8	58.6	994	239	20.8	17.3	3.5
107	Pilchards, canned in tomato sauce	0	70.4	601	144	16.7	8.1	1.7
108	Prawns, boiled	62	70.0	418	99	22.6	0.9	0.2
109	Sardines, canned in oil, drained	18	58.6	918	220	23.3	14.1	2.9
110	Tuna, canned in brine, drained	19	74.6	422	99	23.5	0.6	0.2
111	Salmon, grilled	18	60.7	896	215	24.2	13.1	2.5
	Potato and Potato Products							
112	Chips, homemade, fried in blended oil	0	56.5	796	189	3.9	6.7	0.6
113	French fries, retail	0	43.8	1174	280	3.3	15.5	5.8
114	Oven chips, frozen, baked	0	58.5	687	162	3.2	4.2	1.8
115	Potato crisps	0	2.8	2215	530	5.7	34.2	14.0
116	Potatoes, new, average, boiled in unsalted water	0	80.5	321	75	1.5	0.3	0.1
117	Potatoes, old, average, raw, flesh only	20	79.0	318	75	2.1	0.2	0.0
118	Potatoes, old, baked, flesh and skin	0	62.6	581	136	3.9	0.2	0.0
119	Potatoes, old, boiled in unsalted water	0	80.3	306	72	1.8	0.1	0.0
120	Potatoes, old, roast in blended oil	0	64.7	630	149	2.9	4.5	0.4
	Vegetables							
121	Beans, baked, canned in tomato sauce	0	71.5	355	84	5.2	0.6	0.1
122	Beans, red kidney, canned, drained	36	67.5	424	100	6.9	0.6	0.1
123	Beans, runner, boiled in unsalted water	0	92.8	76	18	1.2	0.5	0.1
124	Beetroot, boiled in salted water	20	82.4	195	46	2.3	0.1	0.0
125	Broccoli, green, raw	39	88.2	138	33	4.4	0.9	0.2
126	Broccoli, boiled in unsalted water	0	91.1	100	24	3.1	0.8	0.2
127	Brussel sprouts, boiled in unsalted water	0	86.9	153	35	2.9	1.3	0.3
128	Cabbage, boiled in unsalted water, average	0	93.1	67	16	1.0	0.4	0.1
129	Cabbage, raw, average	23	90.1	109	26	1.7	0.4	0.1
130	Carrots, old, raw	30	89.8	146	35	0.6	0.3	0.1
131	Carrots, old, boiled in unsalted water	0	90.5	100	24	0.6	0.4	0.1
132	Cauliflower, boiled in unsalted water	0	90.6	117	28	2.9	0.9	0.2
133	Celery, raw	9	95.1	30	7	0.5	0.2	0.0
134	Courgette, boiled in unsalted water	0	93.0	81	19	2.0	0.4	0.1
135	Courgette, fried in corn oil	0	86.8	265	63	2.6	4.8	0.6
136	Cucumber	3	96.4	40	10	0.7	0.1	0.0
137	Hummus	0	61.4	781	187	7.6	12.6	N
138	Lentils, (red dried) boiled in unsalted water	0	72.1	424	100	7.6	0.4	0.0

Carbo-hydrate (g)	Total Sugars (g)	Fibre NSP (g)	Calcium (mg)	Iron (mg)	Sodium (mg)	Vitamin A (µg)	Folate (µg)	Vitamin C (mg)	No.
11.7	0.0	0.5	67	0.5	160	N	57	0	103
16.6	0.0	0.7	92	0.8	440	0	16	0	104
0.0	0.0	0.0	26	0.1	73	0	9	0	105
0.0	0.0	0.0	12	0.8	63	48	N	0	106
1.1	0.9	0.0	250	2.5	290	(30)	N	0	107
0.0	0.0	0.0	110	1.1	1590	0	N	0	108
0.0	0.0	0.0	500	2.3	450	7	8	0	109
0.0	0.0	0.0	8	1.0	320	N	4	0	110
0.0	0.0	0.0	25	0.5	54	16	19	0	111
30.1	0.6	2.2	11	0.8	12	0	43	9	112
34.0	1.3	(2.1)	14	1.0	310	0	31	4	113
29.8	0.7	2.0	(12)	0.8	53	0	21	12	114
53.3	0.7	5.3	29	1.4	800	0	30	35	115
17.8	1.1	1.1	5	0.3	9	0	18	15	116
17.2	0.6	1.3	5	0.4	7	0	35	11	117
31.7	1.2	2.7	11	0.7	12	0	44	14	118
17.0	0.7	1.2	5	0.4	7	0	19	6	119
25.9	0.6	1.8	8	0.7	9	0	36	8	120
15.3	5.9	3.7	53	1.4	530	12	22	0	121
17.8	3.6	6.2	71	2.0	390	1	15	0	122
2.3	2.0	1.9	22	1.0	1	20	42	10	123
9.5	8.8	1.9	29	0.8	110	5	110	5	124
1.8	1.5	2.6	56	1.7	8	96	90	87	125
1.1	0.9	2.3	40	1.0	(13)	79	64	44	126
3.5	3.0	3.1	20	0.5	2	53	110	60	127
2.2	2.0	1.8	33	0.3	8	134	39	20	128
4.1	4.0	2.4	52	0.7	5	192	75	49	129
7.9	7.4	2.4	25	0.3	25	2079	12	6	130
4.9	4.6	2.5	24	0.4	50	2234	16	2	131
2.1	1.8	1.6	17	0.4	4	10	51	27	132
0.9	0.9	1.1	41	0.4	60	8	16	8	133
2.0	1.9	1.2	19	0.6	1	102	31	11	134
2.6	2.5	1.2	38	1.4	1	83	42	15	135
1.5	1.4	0.6	18	0.3	3	10	9	2	136
11.6	1.9	2.4	41	1.9	670	N	N	1	137
17.5	0.8	1.9	16	2.4	12	(3)	33	0	138

Table 3.1 Composition per 100 g of edible portion (continued).

No.	Food	Inedible waste (%)	Water (g)	Energy (kj)	Energy kcal	Protein (g)	Fat (g)	Saturated Fatty Acid (g)
139	Lettuce, average	26	95.1	59	14	0.8	0.5	0.1
140	Mycoprotein, Quorn®	0	74.2	389	92	14.1	3.2	0.6
141	Mushrooms, raw	3	92.6	55	13	1.8	0.5	0.1
142	Onions, raw	9	89.0	150	36	1.2	0.2	0.0
143	Onions, fried in corn oil	0	65.7	684	164	2.3	11.2	1.4
144	Parsnips, boiled in unsalted water	0	78.7	278	66	1.6	1.2	0.2
145	Peas, frozen, boiled in unsalted water	0	78.3	291	69	6.0	0.9	0.2
146	Peas, processed, canned, re-heated, drained	35	69.6	423	99	6.9	0.7	0.1
147	Peppers, green, raw	16	93.3	65	15	0.8	0.3	0.1
148	Plantain, boiled in unsalted water	0	68.5	477	112	0.8	0.2	0.1
149	Spinach, frozen, boiled in unsalted water	0	91.6	90	21	3.1	(0.8)	0.1
150	Swede, boiled in unsalted water	0	95.8	46	11	0.3	0.1	0.0
151	Sweetpotato, boiled in unsalted water	0	74.7	358	84	1.1	0.3	0.1
152	Sweetcorn kernels, canned, re-heated, drained	18	72.3	519	122	2.9	1.2	0.2
153	Tofu, soya bean, steamed	0	85.0	304	73	8.1	4.2	0.5
154	Tomatoes, raw	0	93.1	73	17	0.7	0.3	0.1
155	Turnip, boiled in unsalted water	0	93.1	51	12	0.6	0.2	0.0
156	Vegeburger, retail, grilled	0	50.3	821	196	16.6	11.1	N
157	Watercress	38	92.5	94	22	3.0	1.0	0.3
158	Yam, boiled in unsalted water	0	64.4	568	133	1.7	0.3	0.1
	Fruit							
159	Apples, eating, average, raw, flesh and skin	11	84.5	199	47	0.4	0.1	0.0
160	Apricots, ready-to-eat (semi-dried)	0	29.7	674	158	4.0	0.6	N
161	Avocado, average, flesh only	29	72.5	784	190	1.9	19.5	4.1
162	Bananas, flesh only	34	75.1	403	95	1.2	0.3	0.1
163	Blackcurrants, stewed, with sugar	0	72.9	252	58	0.7	0.0	0.0
164	Cherries, raw, flesh and skin	17	82.8	203	48	0.9	0.1	0.0
165	Dates, raw, flesh and skin	16	14.6	1151	270	3.3	0.2	0.1
166	Figs, ready-to-eat	0	23.6	889	209	3.3	1.5	N
167	Grapefruit, raw, flesh only	32	89.0	126	30	0.8	0.1	0.0
168	Grapes, average	5	81.8	257	60	0.4	0.1	0.0
169	Kiwi fruit, flesh and seeds	14	84.0	207	49	1.1	0.5	N
170	Mangoes, ripe, raw, flesh only	32	82.4	245	57	0.7	0.2	0.1
171	Melon, honeydew, flesh only	37	92.2	119	28	0.6	0.1	0.0
172	Olives, in brine	20	76.5	422	103	0.9	11.0	1.7
173	Oranges, flesh only	30	86.1	158	37	1.1	0.1	0.0
174	Peaches, raw, flesh and skin	10	88.9	142	33	1.0	0.1	0.0
175	Peaches canned in syrup	0	81.1	233	55	0.5	0.0	0.0
176	Peaches, canned in juice	0	86.7	165	39	0.6	0.0	0.0
177	Pears, average, raw, flesh and skin	9	83.8	169	40	0.3	0.1	0.0

Carbo-hydrate (g)	Total Sugars (g)	Fibre NSP (g)	Calcium (mg)	Iron (mg)	Sodium (mg)	Vitamin A (µg)	Folate (µg)	Vitamin C (mg)	No.
1.7	1.7	0.9	28	0.7	3	171	55	5	139
1.9	0.8	4.8	29	0.6	348	0	21	0	140
0.4	0.2	1.1	6	0.6	5	0	44	1	141
7.9	5.6	1.4	25	0.3	3	2	17	5	142
14.1	10.0	3.1	47	0.8	4	7	38	3	143
12.9	5.9	4.7	50	0.6	4	5	41	10	144
9.7	2.7	5.1	35	1.6	2	95	33	12	145
17.5	1.5	4.8	33	1.8	380	10	11	0	146
2.6	2.4	1.6	8	0.4	4	29	36	120	147
28.5	5.5	1.2	5	0.5	4	(58)	22	9	148
0.5	0.3	(2.1)	150	1.7	16	(1101)	52	6	149
2.3	2.2	0.7	26	0.1	14	28	18	15	150
20.5	11.6	2.3	23	0.7	32	660	8	17	151
26.6	9.6	1.4	4	0.5	270	18	20	1	152
0.7	0.3	N	510	1.2	4	0	15	0	153
3.1	3.1	1.0	7	0.5	9	94	22	17	154
2.0	1.9	1.9	45	0.2	28	3	8	10	155
8.0	3.6	4.2	100	4.5	490	N	95	N	156
0.4	0.4	1.5	170	2.2	49	420	45	62	157
33.0	0.7	1.4	12	0.4	17	0	6	4	158
11.8	11.8	1.8	4	0.1	3	3	1	6	159
36.5	36.5	6.3	73	3.4	14	91	11	1	160
1.9	0.5	3.4	11	0.4	6	3	11	6	161
23.2	20.9	1.1	6	0.3	1	4	14	11	162
15.0	15.0	2.8	47	1.0	2	13	N	115	163
11.5	11.5	0.9	13	0.2	1	4	5	11	164
68.0	68.0	4.0	45	1.3	10	7	13	0	165
48.6	48.6	6.9	230	3.9	57	10	8	1	166
6.8	6.8	1.3	23	0.1	3	3	26	36	167
15.4	15.4	0.7	13	0.3	2	3	2	3	168
10.6	10.3	1.9	25	0.4	4	7	N	59	169
14.1	13.8	2.6	12	0.7	2	116	N	37	170
6.6	6.6	0.6	9	0.1	32	8	2	9	171
0.0	0.0	2.9	61	1.0	2250	30	0	0	172
8.5	8.5	1.7	47	0.1	5	8	31	54	173
7.6	7.6	1.5	7	0.4	1	19	3	31	174
14.0	14.0	0.9	3	0.2	4	13	7	5	175
9.7	9.7	0.8	4	0.4	12	11	2	6	176
10.0	10.0	2.2	11	0.2	3	3	2	6	177

Table 3.1 Composition per 100 g of edible portion (continued).

No.	Food	Inedible waste (%)	Water (g)	Energy (kj)	Energy (kcal)	Protein (g)	Fat (g)	Saturated Fatty Acid (g)
178	Pineapple, canned in juice	0	86.8	200	47	0.3	0.0	0.0
179	Plums, average, raw, flesh and skin	6	83.9	155	36	0.6	0.1	0.0
180	Prunes, ready-to-eat	14	31.1	601	141	2.5	0.4	N
181	Raisins	0	13.2	1159	272	2.1	0.4	N
182	Raspberries, raw	0	87.0	109	25	1.4	0.3	0.1
183	Rhubarb, stewed with sugar	0	84.6	203	48	0.9	0.1	0.0
184	Satsumas	29	87.4	155	36	0.9	0.1	0.0
185	Strawberries, raw	5	89.5	113	27	0.8	0.1	0.0
	Nuts							
186	Almonds, flesh only	63	4.2	2534	612	21.1	55.8	4.4
187	Cashew nuts, roasted and salted	0	2.4	2533	611	20.5	50.9	10.1
188	Coconut, desiccated	0	2.3	2492	604	5.6	62.0	53.4
189	Peanut butter, smooth	0	1.1	2510	606	22.6	51.8	12.8
190	Peanuts, roasted and salted	0	1.9	2491	602	24.5	53.0	9.5
	Sugars and preserves							
191	Chocolate, milk	0	1.3	2177	520	7.7	30.7	18.3
192	Honey	0	17.5	1229	288	0.4	0.0	0.0
193	Jam, fruit with edible seeds	0	29.8	1114	261	0.6	0.0	0.0
194	Marmalade	0	28.0	1114	261	0.1	0.0	0.0
195	Peppermints	0	0.2	1678	393	0.5	0.7	N
196	Sugar, white	0	0.0	1680	394	0.0	0.0	0.0
197	Syrup, golden	0	20.0	1269	298	0.3	0.0	0.0
198	Toffee	0	2.4	1793	426	2.2	18.6	9.5
	Beverages							
199	Cocoa powder	0	3.4	1301	312	18.5	21.7	12.8
200	Coffee, infusion, average	0	98.3	8	2	0.2	0.0	0.0
201	Drinking chocolate powder	0	2.1	1582	373	5.4	5.8	3.4
202	Drinking chocolate made up with semi-skimmed milk	0	82.3	310	73	3.6	2.0	1.3
203	Tea, black, infusion, average	0	99.5	0	0	0.1	0.0	0.0
	Soft drinks and juices							
204	Cola	0	89.7	174	41	0.0	0.0	0.0
205	Cola, diet	0	99.8	2	1	0.0	0.0	0.0
206	Lemonade, bottled	0	93.8	93	22	0.0	0.0	0.0
207	Orange juice, unsweetened	0	89.2	153	36	0.5	0.1	0.0
208	Pineapple juice, unsweetened	0	87.8	177	41	0.3	0.1	0.0
209	Fruit drink/squash, undiluted	0	74.4	399	93	0.1	0.0	0.0
210	Fruit juice drink, ready to drink	0	89.5	159	37	0.1	0.0	0.0
211	Fruit juice drink, low calorie, ready to drink	0	96.6	43	10	0.2	0.0	0.0

Carbo-hydrate (g)	Total Sugars (g)	Fibre NSP (g)	Calcium (mg)	Iron (mg)	Sodium (mg)	Vitamin A (μg)	Folate (μg)	Vitamin C (mg)	No.
12.2	12.2	0.5	8	0.5	1	2	1	11	178
8.8	8.8	1.6	13	0.4	?	63	3	4	179
31.0	34.0	5.7	34	2.6	11	23	3	0	180
69.3	69.3	2.0	46	3.8	60	2	10	1	181
4.6	4.6	2.5	25	0.7	3	1	33	32	182
11.5	11.5	1.2	33	0.1	1	5	4	5	183
8.5	8.5	1.3	31	0.1	4	13	33	27	184
6.0	6.0	1.1	16	0.4	6	1	20	77	185
6.9	4.2	(7.4)	240	3.0	14	0	48	0	186
18.8	5.6	3.2	35	6.2	290	1	68	0	187
6.4	6.4	13.7	23	3.6	28	0	9	0	188
13.1	6.7	5.4	37	2.1	350	0	53	0	189
7.1	3.8	6.0	37	1.3	400	0	52	0	190
56.9	56.9	0.8	220	1.4	85	27	11	0	191
76.4	76.4	0.0	5	0.4	11	0	N	0	192
69.0	69.0	N	12	0.2	29	0	0	10	193
69.5	69.5	(0.3)	26	0.2	64	8	5	10	194
102.7	102.7	0.0	7	0.2	9	0	0	0	195
105.0	105.0	0.0	(10)	(0.2)	5	0	0	0	196
79.0	79.0	0.0	16	0.4	270	0	0	0	197
66.7	44.8	0.0	73	0.2	340	0	0	0	198
11.5	0.0	12.1	130	10.5	950	(7)	38	0	199
0.3	0.0	0.0	3	0.1	0	0	0	0	200
79.7	777	N	39	3.5	228	N	7	0	201
10.9	10.7	0.0	114	0.3	58	18	5	1	202
0.0	0.0	0.0	0	0.0	0	0	3	0	203
10.9	10.9	0.0	6	0.0	5	0	0	0	204
0.0	0.0	0.0	(6)	0.0	(5)	0	0	0	205
5.8	5.8	0.0	5	0.0	7	0	0	0	206
8.8	8.8	0.1	10	0.2	10	3	18	39	207
10.5	10.5	0.0	8	0.2	8	1	8	11	208
24.8	24.6	0.0	6	0.0	40	115	2	25	209
9.8	9.8	0.0	6	0.0	5	N	2	23	210
2.5	2.5	0.0	5	0.0	5	0	2	5	211

Table 3.1 Composition per 100 g of edible portion (continued).

No.	Food	Inedible waste (%)	Water (g) (mg)	Energy (kj)	kcal	Protein (g)	Fat (g)	Saturated Fatty Acids (g)
	Miscellaneous							
212	Baking powder	0	6.3	693	163	5.2	0.0	0.0
213	Yeast extract	0	26.7	763	180	40.7	0.4	N
214	Mayonnaise, retail	0	18.0	2843	691	1.1	75.6	11.4
215	Mayonnaise, retail, reduced fat	0	59.5	1188	288	1.0	28.1	4.2
216	Mustard, smooth	0	63.7	579	139	7.1	8.2	0.5
217	Pickle, sweet	0	60.7	604	141	0.6	0.1	0.0
218	Salad cream	0	47.2	1440	348	1.5	31.0	3.3
219	Soup, cream of tomato, canned, ready-to-serve	0	84.2	219	52	0.8	3.0	0.5
220	Soy sauce	0	68.6	182	43	3.0	0.0	0.0
221	Tomato ketchup	0	68.0	489	115	1.6	0.1	0.0
222	French dressing	0	33.3	1902	462	0.1	49.4	8.0
223	Gravy, instant granules, made up	0	93.0	142	34	0.3	2.4	N
224	Pasta sauce, tomato based	0	83.9	200	47	2.0	1.5	0.2
	Alcoholic drinks							
225	Beer, bitter, average	0	93.9	124	30	0.3	0.0	0.0
226	Cider, dry	0	92.5	152	36	0.0	0.0	0.0
227	Lager	0	93.0	121	29	0.3	0.0	0.0
228	Lager, alcohol free	0	96.3	31	7	0.4	0.0	0.0
229	Spirits, 40% volume	0	68.3	919	222	0.0	0.0	0.0
230	Wine, white, medium	0	86.3	308	74	0.1	0.0	0.0
231	Wine, red	0	88.4	283	68	0.1	0.0	0.0

N = Nutrient present in significant quantity but there is no reliable information on the amount.
( ) = Estimated value.

Carbo-hydrate (g)	Total Sugars (g)	Fibre NSP (g)	Calcium (mg)	Iron (mg)	Sodium (mg)	Vitamin A (µg)	Folate (µg)	Vitamin C (mg)	No.
37.8	0.0	0.0	1130	0.0	11800	0	0	U	212
3.5	1.6	0.0	70	2.9	4300	0	2620	0	213
1.7	1.3	0.0	8	0.3	450	103	4	0	214
8.2	4.6	0.0	N	N	(940)	10	N	0	215
9.7	7.8	N	70	2.9	2950	N	0	0	216
36	33.9	1.2	15	0.6	1610	42	0	0	217
16.7	16.7	N	18	0.5	1040	12	3	0	218
5.9	2.6	0.7	17	0.4	400	(75)	12	0	219
8.2	7.3	0.0	17	2.4	7120	0	11	0	220
28.6	27.5	0.9	13	0.3	1630	79	1	2	221
4.5	4.5	0.0	N	N	460	0	0	0	222
3.0	0.1	0.0	1	0.0	460	N	0	0	223
6.9	5.7	N	23	0.7	410	(17)	10	0	224
2.2	2.2	0.0	8	0.1	6	0	5	U	225
2.6	2.6	0.0	8	0.5	7	0	N	0	226
0.0	0.0	0.0	5	0.0	7	0	12	0	227
1.5	1.2	0.0	3	0.0	2	0	5	0	228
0.0	0.0	0.0	0	0.0	0	0	0	0	229
3.0	3.0	0.0	12	0.8	11	0	0	0	230
0.2	0.2	0.0	7	0.9	7	0	1	0	231

Appendix 4   The use of food tables for calculations of the nutritional value of foods

A great deal of useful information can be worked out from the food composition tables in Appendix 3. Examples of various types of calculations are given below:

1. NUTRIENT CONTENT

(a) Simple nutrient content

To calculate the protein content of 2 grilled fish fingers:
Fish fingers (food no. 104) contain 14.3 g protein per 100 g
2 fish fingers weigh 56 g (Appendix 5)

56 g grilled fish fingers contain $14.3 \times \dfrac{56}{100}$

$= 8.0$ g protein

(b) Nutrient content allowing for wastage (inedible matter)

To calculate the carbohydrate content of one apple weighing 120 g:
Eating apples (food no.159) contain 11.8 g carbohydrate per 100 g
edible portion, and 11 per cent waste

A 120 a apple contains $\dfrac{100 - 11}{100} \times 120$ g edible matter

$= 106.8$ g edible matter

Therefore 106.8 g (120 g whole apple) contains x $\dfrac{11.8 \times 106.8}{100}$

$= 12.6$ g carbohydrate

2. PORTION SIZES

(a) 400 kJ portions

Cheddar cheese, for example:
Cheddar cheese (food no. 55) has an energy value of 1725 kJ per 100 g

400 kJ are contained in $\dfrac{100}{1725} \times 400 = 23.2$ g (a little less than 1 oz
Cheddar cheese)

or cottage cheese:

Cottage cheese (food no. 264) has an energy value of 423 kJ per 100 g

400 kJ are contained in $\dfrac{100}{413}$ x 400 = 95 g (or about 3½ oz) of cottage cheese

(b) *100-kcal portions* (the size of a 100-kcal portion will be slightly greater than a 400-kJ portion and slightly smaller than a 500 kJ portion)

Old potatoes, uncooked, for example:

Old potatoes (food no. 117) have an energy value of 75 kcal per 100 g edible portion

100 kcal are contained in $\dfrac{100}{75}$ x 100 = 133 g potato

Since the potatoes contain 20 per cent inedible material (peelings) this is equivalent to

133 x $\dfrac{100}{100 - 20}$ g = 166 g whole potato

3. COST OF NUTRIENTS

(a) *Nutrients per penny*

To calculate the nutrients obtained per penny from a large (800 g) loaf of sliced whole meal bread costing 91p:

1p buys $\dfrac{1}{91}$ x 800 = 8.8 g

Food no. 13 shows the nutrients in 100 g whole meal bread. Therefore multiply the values for each nutrient by $\dfrac{8.8}{100}$ = 0.8 g protein

0.2 g fat
3.7 g carbohydrate
9.3 mg calcium
0.2 mg iron, etc.

(b) To calculate the cost of 10 g protein from *baked beans*

Baked beans (food no. 121) contain 5.2 g protein per 100 g

10 g protein are contained in 10 x $\dfrac{100}{5.2}$ = 192.3 g baked beans

At a cost of 42 p per 420 g can

192.3 g of baked beans cost $\dfrac{192.3}{420}$ x 42 = 19.2 pence

4. PERCENTAGE OF ENERGY FROM FAT

(a) *In a food such as brown bread:*

Brown bread (food no. 9) contains 2.0 g fat and 882 kJ (207 kcal) per 100 g

Each gram of fat provides 37 kJ (9 kcal)

The percentage of energy from fat $= \dfrac{2.0 \times 37}{882} \times 100 = 8.4\%$

$$(\text{or } \dfrac{2.0 \times 9}{207} \times 100 = 8.7\%)$$

(b) Margarine:

Margarine (food no. 67) contains 82.8 g fat and 3067 kJ (746 kcal) per 100 g
Each gram of fat provides 37 kJ (9 kcal)

The percentage of energy from fat $= \dfrac{82.8 \times 37}{3067} \times 100 = 99.9\%$

$$(\text{or } \dfrac{82.8 \times 9}{746} \times 100 = 99.9\%)$$

(c) In a combination of foods:

One slice of brown bread weighs 30 g and 7 g of margarine is allowed for spreading on one slice.
One slice (30 g) brown bread contains

$$(2.0 \times \dfrac{30}{100} \text{ g fat and } (882 \times \dfrac{30}{100}) \text{ kJ}$$

$$= 0.6 \text{ g fat and } 264.6 \text{ kJ (63.2 kcal)}$$

7 g margarine contains $82.8 \times \dfrac{7}{100}$ g fat and $(3067 \times \dfrac{7}{100})$ kJ

$$= 5.8 \text{ g fat and } 214.7 \text{ kJ (51.3 kcal)}$$

The combination slice of bread with margarine contains 0.6 + 5.8 g fat = 6.4 g fat and 264.6 + 214.7 kJ = 479.3 kJ (114.6 kcal)

Since each gram of fat provides 37 kJ or 9 kcal, the percentage of energy from fat in a slice of bread and butter is

$$\dfrac{6.4 \times 37 \times 100}{479.3} = 49.4\%$$

$$(\text{or } \dfrac{6.4 \times 9 \times 100}{114.6} = 50.3\%)$$

Adding baked beans, a banana, or a drink such as fruit juice would further reduce the proportion of energy derived from fat.

N.B. The values derived from kilojoules and kilocalories differ slightly since the conversion factors given on p. 141 are not exactly equivalent.

Appendix 5   Typical servings of commonly used foods

Milk, whole	for 1 cup of tea/coffee	25 g
Milk, semi-skimmed}	for 1 cup of tea/coffee	30 g
	for 1 glass	200 g
Cheese, cheddar type	'matchbox-sized' piece	30 g
Yogurt, plain or fruit	small carton	125 g
Chicken, roast	medium average portion	100 g
Pork chop	medium size, with bone, grilled	150 g
Minced beef	medium average portion, cooked	140 g
Bacon	rasher, average, fried/grilled	40 g
Sausage	large, cooked	40 g
Meat pie	individual pie	150 g
Beefburger, 100% beef	1 burger, fried/grilled	34 g
Fish finger	1 fish finger, grilled	28 g
White fish	medium fillet	150 g
Tuna	1 portion, for sandwich	45 g
Egg	Size 3, no shell	57 g
Baked beans	medium portion	135 g
Butter, margarine or low-fat spread	for 1 slice bread	7-10 g
Oil	1 tablespoon	11 g
Mayonnaise	1 heaped tablespoon	33 g
Peanut butter	thickly spread on 1 slice	20 g
Jam or marmalade	average spreading on 1 slice	15 g
Lettuce	average serving in salad	30 g
Tomato}	1 slice	17 g
	1 medium tomato	85 g
Peas	medium portion	70 g
Carrots	large portion	85 g
Orange	medium-sized, without peel	160 g
Apple	medium-sized, eating	112 g
Banana	1 medium, without skin	100 g
Grapes	small bunch	100 g
Peaches, canned in syrup or juice	average portion	120 g
Raisins/sultanas, dried	1 tablespoon	30 g
Fruit juice	average glass	160 g

Potatoes, boiled	1 average portion, medium	175 g
mashed	1 scoop	60 g
baked,		
with skin	1 medium	180 g
Yam, boiled	size of medium potato	130 g
Bread, whole meal,		
large loaf	medium slice	36 g
Flour	1 tablespoon, rounded	30 g
Porridge	medium portion	160 g
Breakfast cereal}	cornflakes type, medium portion	30 g
	muesli, average, medium portion	50 g
Crispbread	1 crispbread, whole meal	15 g
Biscuits, digestive	1 biscuit	13 g
Rice, boiled	medium portion	180 g
Pasta, cooked	medium portion	230 g
Coffee, instant	1 heaped teaspoon	2 g
Drinking chocolate	per mug	18 g
Sugar	1 level teaspoon	4 g
Beer	half pint	287 g (284 ml)
Wine	1 average glass	25 g (125 ml)

Appendix 6   The eatwell plate

The *eatwell plate* (formerly The Balance of Good Health) forms the basis of the Government's healthy eating advice to the general population. As seen in the illustration opposite, it shows the types and proportions of foods needed to make up a well-balanced, healthy diet. This includes snacks as well as meals. The balance of foods to be achieved is shown by the different areas occupied by each of five food groups: *bread, rice, potatoes, pasta and other starchy foods; fruit and vegetables; meat, fish, eggs, beans and other sources of protein; milk and dairy foods;* and *foods and drinks high in fat and/or sugar.* Choosing food groups in the approximate proportions shown and choosing a variety of different foods from within each group helps to ensure that all essential nutrients are consumed in adequate amounts. People differ in the amount of energy they need and hence in the amount of food they should eat, but whatever that may be the *proportions* of foods from the different groups should remain the same. An individual is therefore advised to look at the plate and try to match the balance in their own diet. The approach recommended is to try and achieve the balance shown every day, but it can also be achieved over the course of a week or so. *The eatwell plate* applies to most people including people whose weight is in the desired range for their height, those who are overweight, vegetarians and people of all ethnic origins. It does not apply to children under two years of age who need full fat milk and dairy products. People under medical supervision or with special dietary requirements should check with their doctor to be clear whether *The eatwell plate* applies to them.

The eatwell plate is accompanied by a set of plate tips that expand the messages conveyed by the diagram:

Try to eat:

- Plenty of fruit and vegetables
- Plenty of bread, rice, potatoes, pasta and other starchy foods – choose wholegrain varieties when you can
- Some milk and dairy foods
- Some meat, fish, eggs, beans and other non-dairy sources of protein
- Just a small amount of foods and drinks high in fat and/or sugar
- Try to choose options that are lower in fat, salt and sugar when you can

A copy of *the eatwell plate* can be obtained from The Food Standards Agency Publications line on 0845 606 0667. Further information on eating a healthy diet is available on www.eatwell.gov.uk

The eatwell plate

Use the eatwell plate to help you get the balance right. It shows how much of what you eat should come from each food group.

FOOD STANDARDS AGENCY
food.gov.uk

Bread, rice, potatoes, pasta and other starchy foods

Milk and dairy foods

Foods and drinks high in fat and/or sugar

Meat, fish, eggs, beans and other non-dairy sources of protein

Fruit and vegetables

Appendix 7   Food additives

In addition to the expected ingredients of made-up foods there are other substances which may be added in small amounts to perform a special function in the food. These are called food additives. They fall into two broad categories: those which are added to prevent food spoilage and those which are added to enhance the texture, flavour or appearance of food.

Preservatives and antioxidants

It is very important that every effort is made to prevent sound food being wasted. Some forms of food spoilage, such as attacks on stored food by vermin, are easily recognised. Other forms of spoilage develop within the food itself and give rise to off-flavours long before the visual appearance of the food itself is noticeably affected; these may arise either by the action of micro-organisms (i.e. moulds and bacteria) or by chemical action. While some microorganisms merely make the food unpalatable, others such as *Clostridium botulinum* produce highly poisonous toxins and present a considerable hazard to health. Preservatives such as sulphur dioxide and sodium nitrite are added to some foods to inhibit the growth of microorganisms. The most common form of chemical spoilage is rancidity. Rancidity resulting from the oxidation of fat can be retarded by the addition of antioxidants. Some antioxidants are natural compounds but in order to protect fat in foods that are baked (e.g. biscuits), heat-stable synthetic antioxidants are required.

Other additives

The texture of food often depends on the ability of added emulsifiers to form a uniform dispersion of fat and water (as in margarine and salad cream). Similarly, stabilisers are added to prevent uniform dispersions separating out (for example, the setting of instant desserts).

The colour and flavour of foods are closely linked: consumers expect a food to have a colour that matches the flavour. Therefore, if the natural colour is lost or changed during processing, colouring matter may be added to restore the food to the expected colour.

The law strictly controls the types and quantities of additives that may be used in food (see also Appendix 8), and the list of ingredients must show the additive category name (e.g. colour), and the serial number of the additive or its name (e.g. E300 ascorbic acid, or E500 sodium bicarbonate) or both.

Appendix 8   Legislation governing the composition and labelling of food

The primary legislation in this field is the Food Safety Act 1990. This extends throughout Great Britain and similar legislation applies in Northern Ireland.

The Act sets out a framework to protect consumers from food being sold which:

(a) is unsafe because it has been rendered injurious to health or is unfit or too contaminated for human consumption;
(b) is not of the nature, substance or quality demanded;
(c) is labelled, advertised or displayed in a manner which falsely describes or misleads.

These general provisions are backed up by many regulations which lay down detailed requirements as to the labelling of all foods, the composition of certain foods, and the type and level of additives and contaminants permitted in food (see below).

The Secretary of State for Health may make legislation having regard to any relevant advice given by the Food Standards Agency. The Secretary of State is required to consult organizations that are representative of interests likely to be affected by such legislative proposals.

The Food Labelling Regulations 1996 require pre-packed foods to bear, amongst other things, its name, a list of ingredients (in descending order by ingoing weight), the name and address of the manufacturer or packer or seller established within the EU and the appropriate indication of durability (a 'use by' or 'best before' date mark) and they include rules on nutrition labelling. Nutrition labelling is compulsory when a nutrition or health claim (e.g. 'low fat', 'helps maintain a health heart') is made, otherwise it can be given voluntarily. When nutrition labelling is given, labels must at the minimum show the amount of energy, protein, carbohydrate and fat provided by 100 g or 100 ml of the food. Per serving or per portion information may be given as well. Some labels show a second group of nutrients which include sugars (as part of carbohydrates), saturates (as part of fat), fibre and sodium. The entire second group has to be added to the basic list if a manufacturer lists or makes a claim about any of them. Labels can also show the amount of polyols (as parts of carbohydrate), starches, monounsaturates, polyunsaturates and cholesterol (as parts of fat) and the amount and percentage of the labelling RDA (a single value is set for food labelling purposes which is sufficient for the needs of the population as a whole) of certain vitamins and minerals, provided the food contains a significant amount. Nutrition information must include the amount of any nutrient if a claim is made about it, including any not already mentioned.

European Regulation 1924/2006 controls the use of nutrition and health claims made on foods. It puts in place a list of authorised nutrition claims that can be made on food and the criteria a product must meet to use them. It also puts in place a process to establish a similar list of health claims, to be completed by January 2010. For a claim to be included or added to the list of health claims, it must be substantiated by supporting scientific evidence that will be assessed by the European Food Safety Authority

Compositional regulations lay down standards for certain foods. For example minimum meat contents are linked to certain permitted names in the Meat Products Regulations. A pork sausage, for instance, under the Meat Products and Spreadable Fish Products Regulations 1984 must contain 65 per cent meat but a beef sausage only 50 per cent.

Certain requirements for the composition of bread are laid down by the Bread and Flour Regulations 1998. The Regulations restrict the use of specified ingredients that may be used in the preparation of flour and bread. The Regulations prescribe the levels of added calcium, iron, thiamin and nicotinic acid required in flour.

The Fruit Juices and Fruit Nectars (England) Regulations 2003 permit the addition of vitamins and minerals to fruit juice and lay down rules on sugar addition. Minimum fruit juice contents are specified for fruit nectars.

The Spreadable Fats (Marketing Standards) Regulations 1995 (as amended) lay down compositional, labelling and marketing standards for spreadable fats (butter, margarine, mixtures and reduced fat spreads) including fortification requirements for vitamins A and D in margarine.

There are also regulations which lay down lists of permitted additives and standards of purity. The safety of additives and the need for their use are given full and detailed consideration before they are permitted to be used in food. Existing regulations control, for example, preservatives, sweeteners, colourings, antioxidants, and emulsifiers and stabilisers. Food contaminants such as heavy metals are also controlled by legislation.

European Regulation 1925/2006 on the addition of vitamins and minerals and certain other substances to food controls which vitamins and minerals can be added to food, the levels added and their purity. It also allows substances, which represent a potential risk to consumers, to be controlled or prohibited.

Details of Regulations pertaining to food are available on the Food Standards Agency web site www.food.gov.uk

Appendix 9   Further reading

Government reviews and reports on nutrition

Department of Health. *Dietary sugars and human disease.* Report on health and social subjects No. 37. London: HMSO, 1989 (0 11 321255 0).

Department of Health. *Dietary Reference Values for food energy and nutrients for the United Kingdom.* Report on health and social subjects No. 41. London: HMSO, 1991 (minor amendments, revised Chapter 36, 1994) (ISBN 0 11 321397 2).

Department of Health. *Dietary Reference Values: a guide.* London: HMSO, 1991 (ISBN 0 11 321396 4).

Department of Health. *The nutrition of elderly people.* Report on health and social subjects No. 43. London: HMSO, 1992 (ISBN 0 11 321550 9).

Department of Health. *Folic acid and the prevention of neural tube defects.* Heywood: Health Publications Unit, 1992.

Department of Health. *The nutritional assessment of novel foods and processes. Report of the Panel on Novel Foods of the Committee on Medical Aspects of Food Policy.* Report on health and social subjects No. 44. London: HMSO, 1993 (ISBN 0 11 321632 7).

Department of Health. *Weaning and the weaning diet.* Report on health and social subjects No. 45. London. HMSO, 1994 (ISBN 0 11 321838 9).

Department of Health. *Nutritional aspects of cardiovascular disease. Report of the Cardiovascular Review Group of the Committee on Medical Aspects of Food Policy.* Report on health and social subjects No. 46. London. HMSO, 1994 (ISBN 0 11 321875 3).

Department of Health. *Nutritional aspects of the development of cancer.* Report on health and social subjects No. 48. London, The Stationery Office, 1998 (ISBN 0 11 322089 8)

Department of Health. *Nutrition and bone health: with particular reference to calcium and vitamin D.* Report on health and social subjects No. 49. London, The Stationery Office, 1998 (ISBN 0 11 322262 9).

K Sproston and P Primatesta. *Health Survey for England 2003.* London, The Stationery Office, 2004.
See also Department of Health web site: www.dh.gov.uk

Scientific Advisory Committee on Nutrition. *Salt and Health.* London, The Stationery Office, 2003 (ISBN 0 11 243075 9).

Scientific Advisory Committee on Nutrition. *Advice on fish consumption: benefits and risks.* London. The Stationery Office, 2004 (ISBN 0 11 243083 X).

Scientific Advisory Committee on Nutrition. *Review of Dietary Advice on Vitamin A.* London, The Stationery Office, 2005 (ISBN 0 11 243088 0).

Scientific Advisory Committee on Nutrition. *Folate and disease prevention.* London. The Stationery Office, 2006 (ISBN 0 11 243111 9).

Scientific Advisory Committee on Nutrition. *Update on vitamin D. Position Statement by the SACN.* London. The Stationery Office, 2007 (ISBN 978 0 11 243114 5) See also SACN web site: www.sacn.gov.uk

Report on safety aspects of nutrients
Expert Group on Vitamins and Minerals. *Safe Upper Levels for Vitamins and Minerals.* Food Standards Agency, 2003 (ISBN 1 904026 11 7). See: www.food.gov.uk/multimedia/pdfs/vitmin2003.pdf

Government dietary and nutrition surveys
J R Gregory, D L Collins, P S W Davies, J M Hughes and P C Clarke. *National Diet and Nutrition Survey: children aged 1½ to 4½ years. Volume 1: Report of the diet and nutrition survey.* London: HMSO, 1995 (ISBN 0 11 691611 7).

K Hinds and J R Gregory. *National Diet and Nutrition Survey: children aged 1½ to 4½ years. Volume 2: Report of the dental survey.* London: HMSO, 1995 (ISBN 0 11 691612 5).

S Finch, W Doyle, C Lowe, C Bates, A Prentice, G Smithers, P Clarke. *National Diet and Nutrition Survey: people aged 65 years and over. Volume 1: Report of the diet and nutrition survey.* London: The Stationery Office, 1998 (ISBN 0 11 243019 8).

J Steele, A Sheiham, W Marcenes, A Walls. *National Diet and Nutrition Survey: people aged 65 years and over. Volume 2: Report of the oral health survey.* London: The Stationery Office, 1998 (ISBN 0 11 243017 9).

J Gregory, S Lowe et al. *National Diet and Nutrition Survey: young people aged 4 to 18 years. Volume 1. Report of the diet and nutrition survey.* London, The Stationery Office, 2000 (ISBN 0 11 6212659).

L Henderson, J Gregory, K Irving, G Swan. *The National Diet and Nutriiton Survey: adults aged 19 to 64 years. Energy, protein, carbohydrate, fat and alcohol intake.* London, The Stationery Office, 2003. (ISBN 0 11 621567 4).

L Henderson, K Irving et al. *The National Diet and Nutrition Survey: adults aged 19 to 64 years. Vitamin and mineral intake and urinary analytes.* London, The Stationery Office, 2003 (ISBN 0 11 621568 2).

Department of Food and Rural Affairs. *Family Food - A report on the 2003/04 Expenditure and Food Survey.* London, The Stationery Office, 2005.

M Nelson, B Erens, B Bates, S Church, T Boshier. *Low Income Diet and Nutrition Survey.* Vol 1. *Background; methods; sample characteristics.* Vol 2. *Food consumption; nutrient intake.* Vol 3. *Nutritional status; physical activity; economic, social and other factors.* London. The Stationery Office, 2007 (ISBN 978 0 11 703783 0).

Food composition tables
Food Standards Agency. *McCance and Widdowson's The Composition of Foods, Sixth summary edition.* Cambridge: Royal Society of Chemistry, 2002 (ISBN 0 85404 428 0).

Supplements to McCance and Widdowson's The Composition of Foods:
A A Paul, D A T Southgate and J Russell. *Amino acids, mg per 100 g food, fatty acids g per 100 g food.* The first supplement to *McCance and Widdowson's The Composition of Foods.* London: HMSO, 1980 (ISBN 0 444 80220 7).

S P Tan, R W Wenlock and D H Buss. *Immigrant foods.* The second supplement to *McCance and Widdowson's The Composition of Foods* (4th ed.). London: HMSO, 1985 (ISBN 0 11 242717 0).

B Holland, I D Unwin and D H Buss. *Cereals and cereal products.* The third supplement to *McCance and Widdowson's The Composition of Foods* (4th ed.). Nottingham: The Royal Society of Chemistry, 1988 (ISBN 0 85186 743 X).

B Holland, I D Unwin and D H Buss. *Milk products and eggs.* The fourth supplement to *McCance and Widdowson's The Composition of Foods* (4th ed.). Cambridge: The Royal Society of Chemistry, 1989 (ISBN 0 85186 366 3).

B Holland, I D Unwin and D H Buss. *Vegetables, herbs and spices.* The fifth supplement to *McCance and Widdowson's The Composition of Foods* (4th ed.). Cambridge: The Royal Society of Chemistry, 1991 (ISBN 0 85186 376 0).

B Holland, I D Unwin and D H Buss. *Fruit and nuts.* The first supplement to *McCance and Widdowson's The Composition of Foods* (5th ed.). Cambridge: The Royal Society of Chemistry, 1992 (ISBN 0 85186 386 8).

B Holland, A A Welch and D H Buss. *Vegetable dishes.* The second supplement to *McCance and Widdowson's The Composition of Foods* (5th ed.). Cambridge: The Royal Society of Chemistry, 1992 (ISBN 0 85186 396 5).

B Holland, J Brown and D H Buss. *Fish and fish products.* The third supplement to *McCance and Widdowson's The Composition of Foods* (5th ed.). Cambridge: The Royal Society of Chemistry, 1993 (ISBN 085186 421 X).

W Chan, J Brown and D H Buss. *Miscellaneous foods.* The fourth supplement to *McCance and Widdowson's The Composition of Foods* (5th ed.). Cambridge: The Royal Society of Chemistry, 1994 (ISBN 0 85186 360 4).

W Chan, J Brown, S M Lee and D H Buss. Meat, poultry and game. The fifth supplement to *McCance and Widdowson's The Composition of Foods* (5th ed.), Cambridge: The Royal Society of Chemistry, 1995 (ISBN 0 85186 380 9).

W Chan, J Brown, S M Church and D H Buss. Meat products and dishes. The sixth supplement to *McCance and Widdowson's The Composition of Foods* (5th ed.), Cambridge: The Royal Society of Chemistry, 1996 (ISBN 0 85404 809 X).

Ministry of Agriculture, Fisheries and Food. *Fatty acids*. The seventh supplement to *McCance and Widdowson's The Composition of Foods* (5th ed.) Cambridge: The Royal Society of Chemistry, 1998 (ISBN 0 85404 819 7).

Food Portion sizes
Ministry of Agriculture, Fisheries & Food. *Food portion sizes*. London: The Stationery Office, 1993 (2nd ed.) (ISBN 0 11 242961 0).

M Nelson, M Atkinson, J Meyer. *Food Portion Sizes: A Photographic Atlas*. MAFF, 1997.

Policy
Department of Health. *The NHS Cancer Plan*. Department of Health, 2000.
Food Standards Agency Wales. *Food and wellbeing. Reducing inequalities through a nutrition strategy for Wales*. FSAW, 2003.

Department of Health. *Choosing health. Making healthier choices easier*. White Paper. The Stationery Office, 2004.

Department of Health, Social Services and Public Safety. *A healthier future: a 20 year vision for health and wellbeing in Northern Ireland 2005 2025*. DHSSPS, 2004.
Scottish Executive. *Eating for health – meeting the challenge: coordinated action, improved communication and leadership for Scottish Food and Health Policy*. 2004.

Department of Health. *Choosing a better diet: a food and health action plan*. Department of Health Publication, London, 2005.
Healthy Start see www.dh.gov.uk

Department of Health and Department for Children, Schools and Families. *Healthy Weight, Healthy Lives: A Cross Government Strategy for England*. HM Government 2008.

Research
Results of on-going and completed research into the effectiveness of healthy eating interventions with various population groups and settings carried out under the Food Standards Agency's Food Acceptability and Choice Research Programme are on www.food.gov.uk

Healthy eating advice

Advice and guidance on healthier eating for caterers, schools (including vending, tuckshops, cooking clubs, guidance for school governors) and for the public are available on the Food Standards Agency web sites www.food.gov.uk and www.eatwell.gov.uk

Advice on salt is available on www.salt.gov.uk

Advice for schools on a whole school approach to healthy eating is available on www.healthyschools.gov.uk, www.teachernet.gov.uk and www.governet.gov.uk

Advice for caterers of school food is available on the Department for Children, Schools and Families web site www.dcsf.gov.uk and School Food Trust website www.schoolfoodtrust.org.uk for parents on www.parentscentre.gov.uk

Advice for parents on feeding babies and infants 'Birth to Five' is available on www.dh.gov.uk

Advice on healthy eating for babies and children, and on school food, in Welsh is available on www.direct.gov.uk

General reading

J C Drummond and A Wilbraham. *The Fnglishman's food*. London: Pimlico, 1991.

C Geisler and H Powers (eds). *Human nutrition*. 11th edition: Elsevier, 2005 (ISBN 0 443 07356 2).

Index

Page numbers in **bold** type indicate main entries; those in *italics* indicate tables and entries in tables (including any notes). The suffix 'n' indicates a footnote, and 'fig' a figure or diagram.

absorption 34, **38-9**
     minerals 44, 46, 49, 52, 69, 71, 72, 73, 102
acesulfame K 6
acetic acid 32
activity levels and energy expenditure 26-9, *27, 28*, 30
additives 6, 105, **165**
adipose tissue (body fat) 1, 29, 32, 39-40
adolescents 47, 72, 81, **126-7**
alanine 20
alcohol 2, 17, 32, 33, 38, **112**
     alcoholism and heavy drinking 61, 112, 113, 115
     safe drinking levels 128
     wine and spirits 3, *9, 33, 45*, 112, *112*, 162
     see also beers and lagers
allergies and allergens 22-3, 124-5, 133-4
alpha-carotene *60*
alpha-linolenic acid 14, 17
alpha-tocopherol 74, 74n
amino acids 1, 20-1, 22, 23, 42, 64, 65
     cooking and industrial processing 23, 92, *93*, 95
     digestion and absorption 37, *37*, 38, 40
amylase 37, *37*
amylopectin 6
amylose 6
anaemias 4, 44, 66, 67, 74, 132
anencephaly 67
animal fats 12, *13*, 14, 15, *16*
animal proteins 21, 23, *24*
anorexia nervosa 32
anthocyanins 3
antibodies 22, 38
antioxidants 3, 56, 58, 69, 74, **75**, 165
AOAC (Association of Analytical Chemists) method, fibre values 11, *11*
appetite and hunger 34, 80, 99, 125, 126, 129
'apple' shapes 30
arachidonic acid 14

galactose 5, 6, 37, *37*
gall bladder 35fig, 37
gamma linolenic acid (GLA) 14
gas, intestinal 37, 38
gastric juice 36, 66, 99
gastro-intestinal (digestive) tract 34-9
gelatin 23
ghee 97
GI (Glycaemic Index) 133
GLA (gamma linolenic acid) 14
glucose 5, 6, 7, 8, 34, 37, *37*, 39, 40, 54
glucose syrups (liquid glucose) 5, 8, 10, 23, 112
glutamic acid 20
glutamine 20
gluten 22, 23, 104, 105, 124, 133
Glycaemic Index (GI) 133
glycerol (glycerine) 12, 13n
glycine 20
glycogen 7, *37*, 39
goitre 54, 55
'grazing' 114

haem iron 44
haemoglobin 42, 43, 65
hard fats 12, *13*, 14, *16*
HDL (high-density lipoprotein) cholesterol 17
health problems 113
        see also specific problems (e.g. stroke)
healthy diet *see* balanced diet
heart and cardiovascular disease 3, 17-18, 29, 30, 49, 50, 52, 75, 79, 100, 113, 115, 129, 132
heat, effect on nutrients *see* cooking; industrial processing; sunlight
height to weight ratio chart 31fig
high blood pressure 17, 29, 46, 49, 50, 52, 82, 113, 132
high-density lipoprotein (HDL) cholesterol 17
'high fructose' syrups 5
high pressure processing (HPP) 91
High Temperature Short Time (HTST method) 95-6
histidine 20
homogenised milk 95
honey 5, 8, *9*, 10, 81, 112
hormones 2n, 39, 40, 54
HPP (high pressure processing) 91
HTST (High Temperature Short Time) method 95-6
hunger *see* appetite and hunger

hydrochloric acid 36
hydrogenation of fats 12, 18
hypertension *see* high blood pressure

ice cream 8, *9*, *16*, 29, *47*, **97**, *146-7*
ileum 35fig, 36, 38
illnesses 113
    see also specific illnesses (e.g. stroke)
imperial/metric measurements 4, 141
indigestion 38
indispensable amino acids 20, 21
industrial processing **91**, *93*
    effect on starch 7, 104
    emulsification 15
    role of sugars 5, 6, 8
    salt content, processed foods 49-50, 96, 97, 122, 125
    see also cooking; specific foods (e.g. milk)
inedible waste 116, 120, *120*, 143, *144-57*, 158
infants and children **124-6**
    BMR, EAR and energy requirements 25, *26*, *28-9*, *77*, 79, 81, 122, 125-6
    breakfast 115
    breastfeeding *see* lactation and breastfeeding
    cow's milk suitability 6, 43, 47, 48, 54, 70, 95
    digestion 37-8, *37*
    DRVs 79
    five a day fruit and vegetables 108
    foods to avoid 69n, 101, 102, 111
    formula milks 50, 74, *77*, *78*, 124
    macronutrient requirements 4, 20, 22, 78, 81, 122
    mineral requirements 43, 44, 45, 47, 48, 49, 50, 54, *78*, 81, 82, 125
    RNIs *78*
    salt intake 50, 82, 125, 126
    vitamin drops 83, 125
    vitamin requirements 70, 72, 73, 74, *78*, 83, 125-6, 132
    weaning and introducing solids 124-5
ingredients lists 165
insoluble fibre 3, 7
insulin 39, 40
insulin-dependent diabetes *see* diabetes
intense sweeteners 6
intestines 35fig, 36-9, *37*
intrinsic factor 36, 38, 66
intrinsic sugars 10, *79*, 81, 110
invisible fats 12

NSP (non-starch polysaccharides) 5, 7, 10, *11*, 79, *79*, 81, *88-9*, 122, *144-57*
    see also fibre
NTDs (neural tube defects) 67, 82, 129
nutrients
    definition 1, 2
    types 1-2
nutrition, definition 1
nutritional importance, definition 87
nutritional labelling 11, 84, 122, 166-7
nutritional values, calculations and examples 115-21, *117-20*, 158-60
nuts and peanuts **102-3**
    allergies 22-3, 124-5, 133
    average diet *88-9*
    inedible waste 116, 120, *120, 154*
    macronutrients and fibre *11, 13, 16*, 20, *21*, 22, 23, *24*, 103, *154-5*
    minerals *47, 48*, 50, *51*, 53, 54, 55, 56, *155*
    vitamins *62*, 65, *68*, 74, 103, *155*

oats 7, *11*, 15, *16, 24*, 55, 65, 69, 103, 106, 162
obesity 4, 17, **29-31**, 80, 113, 126
oesophagus 35fig
offal *see* liver; meat and meat products
oils 12, *13*, 14, 15, *16*, 18, *33*, 74, 111, *148-9*
    fish liver oils 16, 58, 59, *60*, 73, 100-1, 130
oilseeds 14, 15, 111
oily fish *see* fish
older and elderly people **129-30**
    BMR and energy requirements 25, *26*, 28, *77*, 129
    foods to avoid 69n, 102, 130
    minerals 46, 49, 52, 55, *78*
    RNIs *78*, 84
    vitamins 46, 58, 66, 67, 70, 72, 73, *78*, 82, 83, 130
oleic acid 14
omega-3 and omega-6 polyunsaturated fatty acids 14, 15, 16, 18, 100, 101, 127
organic foods 131-2
osteomalacia 45-6, 72
osteoporosis 46, 58, 82, 130
oxalate 46
oysters 91

PAL (physical activity level) 26-8, 80
palatability 29, 34, 112, 129
palmitic acid 12
pancreas 35fig, 37, *37*